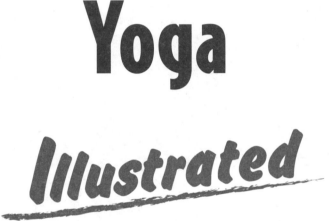

THE COMPLETE IDIOT'S GUIDE® TO

Yoga

Illustrated

Fourth Edition

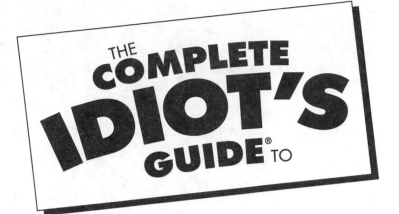

THE COMPLETE IDIOT'S GUIDE® TO

Yoga

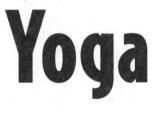

Illustrated

Fourth Edition

by Joan Budilovsky and Eve Adamson
Revised with Carolyn Flynn

ALPHA

A member of Penguin Group (USA) Inc.

This book is dedicated to all yoga students who learn
to teach and teach to learn.
—Joan Budilovsky

ALPHA BOOKS

Published by the Penguin Group

Penguin Group (USA) Inc., 375 Hudson Street, New York, New York 10014, U.S.A.

Penguin Group (Canada), 10 Alcorn Avenue, Toronto, Ontario, Canada M4V 3B2 (a division of Pearson Penguin Canada Inc.)

Penguin Books Ltd, 80 Strand, London WC2R 0RL, England

Penguin Ireland, 25 St Stephen's Green, Dublin 2, Ireland (a division of Penguin Books Ltd)

Penguin Group (Australia), 250 Camberwell Road, Camberwell, Victoria 3124, Australia (a division of Pearson Australia Group Pty Ltd)

Penguin Books India Pvt Ltd, 11 Community Centre, Panchsheel Park, New Delhi—110 017, India

Penguin Group (NZ), cnr Airborne and Rosedale Roads, Albany, Auckland 1310, New Zealand (a division of Pearson New Zealand Ltd)

Penguin Books (South Africa) (Pty) Ltd, 24 Sturdee Avenue, Rosebank, Johannesburg 2196, South Africa

Penguin Books Ltd, Registered Offices: 80 Strand, London WC2R 0RL, England

International Standard Book Number: 1-59257-488-2
Library of Congress Catalog Card Number: 2005937485

08 07 06   8 7 6 5 4 3 2 1

Interpretation of the printing code: The rightmost number of the first series of numbers is the year of the book's printing; the rightmost number of the second series of numbers is the number of the book's printing. For example, a printing code of 06-1 shows that the first printing occurred in 2006.

Printed in the United States of America

Note: This publication contains the opinions and ideas of its authors. It is intended to provide helpful and informative material on the subject matter covered. It is sold with the understanding that the authors, book producer, and publisher are not engaged in rendering professional services in the book. If the reader requires personal assistance or advice, a competent professional should be consulted.

The authors, book producer, and publisher specifically disclaim any responsibility for any liability, loss, or risk, personal or otherwise, which is incurred as a consequence, directly or indirectly, of the use and application of any of the contents of this book.

Most Alpha books are available at special quantity discounts for bulk purchases for sales promotions, premiums, fund-raising, or educational use. Special books, or book excerpts, can also be created to fit specific needs.

For details, write: Special Markets, Alpha Books, 375 Hudson Street, New York, NY 10014.

Publisher: *Marie Butler-Knight*
Editorial Director/Acquiring Editor: *Mike Sanders*
Senior Managing Editor: *Jennifer Bowles*
Book Producer: *Lee Ann Chearney/Amaranth Illuminare*
Development Editor: *Lynn Northrup*
Production Editor: *Megan Douglass*
Copy Editor: *Emily Bell*

Cartoonist: *Shannon Wheeler*
Illustrator: *Wendy Frost*
Book Designer: *Trina Wurst*
Cover Designer: *Bill Thomas*
Indexer: *Angie Bess*
Layout: *Becky Harmon*
Proofreading: *John Etchison*

Contents at a Glance

Contents

Foreword

The world-famous violinist Sir Yehudi Menuhin said about yoga that it is "a technique ideally suited to prevent physical and mental illness and to protect the body generally, developing an inevitable sense of self-reliance and assurance." Yoga did not make him a musical genius, but gave him energy, balance, and a sense of well-being for the last half of his life, allowing him full expression of his great talent.

Yoga can do the same for anyone. Old or young. Male or female. Busy or super-busy. In fact, yoga in one form or another is practiced by several million people today. It has been part of the kaleidoscope of our Western culture for more than a century now and has proven incredibly effective in the maintenance of a sound body and mind and even the restoration of one's health. This is why several progressive insurance companies are now including yoga in their alternative therapies coverage.

Yoga is a tradition that looks back upon at least 5,000 years of experience and experimentation. Although it was created in India in a different cultural environment, the basic insights and laws on which it is based are valid anywhere in the world. Of course, there is much more to yoga than its potency as a system of health care. But this is for you to discover.

In *The Complete Idiot's Guide to Yoga Illustrated, Fourth Edition*, you will be gently but persuasively guided into the beginnings of yoga practice. The authors serve as knowledgeable and cheerful friends, motivating you all the way. Within these pages you will find no lack of encouragement, and everything is explained step by step. So please, take the leap into what you will discover to be a rewarding and healing experience.

Georg Feuerstein, Ph.D., M. Litt.

Georg Feuerstein, Ph.D., M. Litt., is director of the Yoga Research Center; author of *Shambhala Encyclopedia of Yoga* and *Shambhala Guide to Yoga;* and a contributing editor of *Yoga Journal.*

Introduction

Imagine waking up one morning to find that all the stresses in your life have been replaced with total joy. Yes, joy—the kind of pure joy you felt as a child when it was summer and the sun was shining and you had nothing to do but explore the whole world. Now, imagine possessing a strong, flexible body over which you have complete control. To top that off (literally!), imagine a mind free of chaotic thought, confusion, and uncertainty. Imagine pure health, pure consciousness, and pure bliss. This is the realm of the yogi.

And that yogi is you! Even if this realm seems far away now, you will soon be on an amazing journey. We have each traveled down our own yoga paths a little way. We've looked ahead, peeked over the horizon of the next few hills, and now we'd like to give you some hints about how to make the most of what's in store for you on your journey into your self. Yoga is a process of self-discovery, and everyone's discoveries will be different, but we hope to steer you toward the potential "you," the perfect "you," the "you" waiting to be set free.

It won't be difficult. Yoga is beautifully simple. In fact, we think you're gonna love it!

How to Use This Book

This book is divided into five parts, each bringing yoga into your life in a different way.

Part 1, "Let's Do Hatha Yoga," eases you into the concepts of yoga and gets you set up for yoga practice. We talk about why this ancient Eastern system of health has become such a hit with modern Westerners and how yoga can improve all aspects of your fitness, including your performance in other sports. We'll give you a taste of Hatha Yoga, the most popular form of yoga in the West. And we'll give you advice on finding a yoga teacher, buying clothes and equipment, and scheduling yoga into your busy day.

Part 2, "Strength: Poses to Build Endurance," is the first part of exercises. We show you wonderful standing postures, beautiful backbends, terrific twists, and inversions, including the famous headstand posture.

Part 3, "Calm: Poses to Quiet the Body and Mind," is the part of calming and centering postures, including sitting and meditative poses, breathing exercises, forward bends, mudras (meditation hand positions), and mantras (centering chants). We'll devote one chapter to a detailed discussion of shavasana, or Corpse pose, one the most important poses in yoga.

Part 4, "Living Yoga," is all about the yoga lifestyle. We'll show you how to practice yoga with a partner, whether a friend, your life partner, or your child. You can even practice yoga with your whole family! You'll learn why yoga is great for all the stages in a woman's life, from PMS to menopause. You'll learn how yoga can ease life's aches and pains, as well as guide you through more serious illnesses.

Part 5, "Yoga Sessions," will bring you sequences of yoga poses you can use in your practice. We'll start with vinyasana, dynamic combinations of postures that will have you breaking a sweat. Then we'll give you some 5-minute yoga sessions and 15-minute yoga sessions for when you only have a little time, and a sample 30-minute and 60-minute yoga session for when you've got more time to spend.

In Appendix A, you'll get a taste for Joan Budilovsky's yoga column, Yo Joan, which can be found at Yoyoga.com. We have provided a guide to the chakras, or energy centers in the body, in Appendix B. Appendix C provides a glossary of terms, while Appendix D gives some suggestions for further reading.

Yoga Jewels

Throughout this book, we've added four types of extra information in boxes for your enlightenment:

Know Your Sanskrit _____
These boxes give you definitions for Sanskrit (the classical language of India) terms and correct pronunciations, too, so you can talk the talk.

A Yoga Minute _____
These boxes are full of fun anecdotes, trivia, and miscellaneous info about the fascinating world of yoga.

Ouch! _____
These cautionary boxes contain information about how to avoid potential problems.

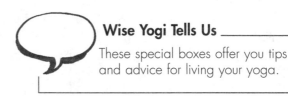

Wise Yogi Tells Us _____
These special boxes offer you tips and advice for living your yoga.

Acknowledgments

Far more people than can ever be mentioned here have, directly or indirectly, helped to make this book what it is. We'll name a few, but we send sincere and grateful energy out to all of you: Joan's dear friend and webmaster Kathie Huddleston, who convinced Joan that she needed a yoga website, and who consequently created the most beautiful Yoyoga! website (www.yoyoga.com). Joan thanks Tom Holoubek for his vibrantly colored photos and Chuck Reiter for his ever-colorful capers. Joan's soulmate, Ben, who inspires her daily in more ways than she can count. Eve's children, Angus and Emmett, who are even more accomplished yogis than they were when this book first came out. Joan's foster children, who, however briefly they hold the key to her home, will forever hold the key to her heart. Eve's dog, Sally, and Joan's cat, Mufasa, for their regular reinforcement of yoga poses at home. Dr. Georg Feuerstein, for his invaluable advice and counsel. Wendy Frost, for her beautiful illustrations that have magnificently expanded with each edition of this book. Carolyn Flynn, for her careful attention to detail in the editing of this fourth edition. Lee Ann Chearney at Amaranth Illuminare, our book producer, for always giving us "all the best," and always promising "more soon!" We amore you, LAC!

The whole team at Alpha Books: Marie Butler-Knight, Mike Sanders, Jen Bowles, and Megan Douglass; our copy editor, Emily Bell; and our development editor, the ever-fabulous Lynn Northrup.

Eve's two favorite yoga teachers in Iowa City, Joyce and Kelli, and her yoga buddy (and buddy otherwise), Lois, who comes along despite her wrists. Joan's beautiful twin sister, Jane, who since birth has been the deeply felt "THA!" in Joan's "HA!" The many wonderful bookstores (the people in them, really) who have encouraged both of us as writers. Joan's parents, John and Leona, and Eve's parents, Richard and Penny. Joan wishes to thank Eve, and Eve wishes to thank Joan, and both of us wish to thank our families and friends who have been there or are there to lend an ear, a hand, a good thought, the right words, or whatever it takes—offering yet another view of the many limbs of yoga.

Special Thanks to the Technical Reviewer

Previous editions of *The Complete Idiot's Guide to Yoga Illustrated* were reviewed by an expert who checked the technical accuracy of what you'll learn here, to help us ensure that this book gives you everything you need to know about yoga. Special thanks are extended to William Hunt.

William Hunt is a certified yoga instructor, ordained priest, and the director of the Hatha Yoga teacher's training program at the Temple of Kriya Yoga in Chicago. He also co-teaches with Dr. Bruno Cortis, cardiologist, in wellness seminars.

Special Thanks to the Book Producer

This book would not have been possible without the expert vision and editorial guidance of Lee Ann Chearney of Amaranth Illuminare. The team at Alpha is immeasurably grateful to her for her hard work and diligence. Thanks, Lee Ann!

Trademarks

All terms mentioned in this book that are known to be or are suspected of being trademarks or service marks have been appropriately capitalized. Alpha Books and Penguin Group (USA) Inc. cannot attest to the accuracy of this information. Use of a term in this book should not be regarded as affecting the validity of any trademark or service mark.

In This Part

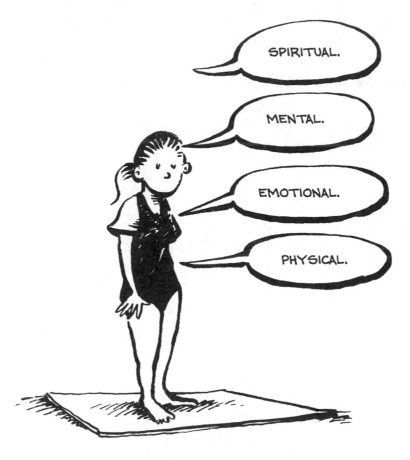

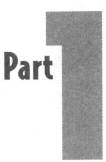

Part 1

Let's Do Hatha Yoga

Yoga is more popular than ever. In Part 1, we'll introduce you to this ancient and venerable system of living and show you why it's relevant, not just for your physical fitness, but for your emotional, mental, and spiritual well-being, too. And the wonderful thing about yoga is that it works, no matter your fitness level, no matter your personal philosophy, no matter your spiritual belief system.

We'll start with Hatha Yoga, the style that is most popular in the West. You'll find out how to get started and develop a routine that increases your strength, flexibility, balance, grace, and muscle tone.

In This Chapter

- ◆ Everybody's doing yoga
- ◆ Yoga mind benefits
- ◆ Yoga body basics
- ◆ More than a fitness program
- ◆ Hatha Yoga's bodymind connection

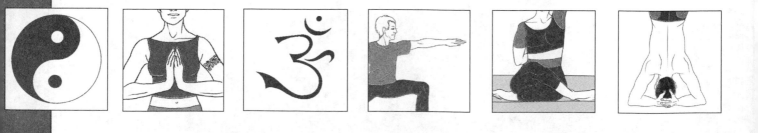

Chapter 1

Yoga Union: Body and Mind Together

Perhaps you have seen those strong, slim, toned, graceful people heading off to yoga class with their brightly colored mats, and you've wondered what this yoga thing is all about. You notice they seem happy, too. They are the people who radiate confidence and contentment. Whether you already are active—involved in a sport or doing some form of regular exercise— or you're a wishful wanna-be, the appeal of yoga certainly has caught your notice.

If so, you aren't alone. Yoga has enjoyed such a surge of interest in the past decade that classes are popping up everywhere. Yoga is a life-empowering system of wholeness and fitness that originated in India. It is a journey of the body and mind, and it can fit into a wide range of personal and fitness goals.

What Is Yoga?

Yoga is mainstream. No longer is it solely the province of those who meditate with Eastern Indian gurus, nor is it athletics "lite." *Yoga Journal* estimates 16.5 million people in the United States practice yoga, while other wellness sociologists say the number could be as high as 28 million. The number of fitness facilities in the United States offering yoga classes surged from 31 percent in 1996 to 85 percent in 2002, as reported by IDEA Health and Fitness Association.

Yoga is a whole-body and whole-mind fitness plan. It flexes your spirit along with your muscles. The poses in yoga, called *asanas*, are designed to work your whole body, not just a few isolated muscle groups. Yoga builds flexibility, strength, balance, and confidence at the same time it improves cardiovascular health, boosts immunity, and optimizes organ function. Some people call it "internal massage." But more than that, practicing yoga's poses helps to nurture the movement of *prana*, the universal life force. Prana is the soul of the universe. Doing yoga maximizes the flow of the universal life force within your body, giving you better health and increased vitality. May the force be with you as you begin doing yoga.

Most of the poses, such as the twists and inversions, stimulate particular internal organs or release energy from stress-prone areas such as the lower back or neck. While other forms of exercise target fat-burning, strength-building, or cardiovascular health, yoga's fine-tuning exercises are the ultimate full-body workout. Yoga does it all.

Although there are many types of yoga, *Hatha Yoga* is the branch of yoga that concentrates on the body and the one most Westerners practice. There are many different styles or approaches of Hatha Yoga that are taught. If one style does not appeal to you, another may. For example, you may enjoy a sweaty aerobic workout (Bikram), or a more relaxed and gentle approach (Sivananda). The *asanas* and philosophy of Hatha Yoga will be the emphasis of this book. *Ha* means "sun," and *tha* means "moon," so *Hatha* is a combining of complementary forces.

Know Your Sanskrit

Yoga (*YOH-gah*) is derived from the Sanskrit root yuj, meaning "to yoke or join together." **Asanas** (*AH-sah-nahs*) are the poses, or exercises, of yoga designed to facilitate meditation. A central concept to yoga is **prana** (*PRAH-nah*), a form of energy in the universe that animates all physical matter, including the human body. **Hatha** (*HATH-a*) **Yoga** is the branch of yoga that transforms the human body via physical strengthening and purification to make the body a worthy vehicle of self-realization.

Body Benefits

Whether you are a beginner or an advanced practitioner, you can gain immediate benefits from yoga. That's because it combines so many different fitness elements and is so easily tailored to the individual. Here's a closer look at the body benefits of yoga:

- Yoga will tone your muscles and trim excess weight. It might even change your attitude about your body for the better.

- Yoga will improve your flexibility. If you're about as flexible as a steel pole, start slowly and go as far into a pose as you can. Every day of practice will take you further.

- Yoga will improve your balance. Standing poses will challenge you to achieve keen muscle control, flexible joints, and great concentration.

- Yoga will make you strong. Yoga draws on isometric training, where muscles are tensed in opposition to each other, but it's much more interesting than calisthenics in high school gym class!

- Yoga will give you the gift of boundless energy. That's because it stimulates your circulatory system and improves organ function—including the brain. You'll feel so much vitality that it seems you gained hours in your day.

- Yoga will help ease your aches, pains, and stiffness. You'll feel like a kid again.

The Learning Curve

Yoga is also user friendly. It doesn't require a lot of equipment, and you don't need to be an expert.

Yoga doesn't hurt. You go at your own pace, do what feels good, and stop before you feel pain. What could be better?

You can do as much or as little yoga as you like. Start with the postures, and you might find that your interest in breathing, chanting, and meditation develops later—or not at all, which is fine, too. It's all up to you.

Anyone can do yoga. It's just a matter of starting at the appropriate level and remembering that you aren't competing with anyone.

> **Wise Yogi Tells Us** _____
> If you are overweight or have a problem with overeating, yoga postures are the perfect exercise for you; they're gentle on stiff joints and can gently condition unconditioned bodies, too! Talk to your doctor about starting an appropriate fitness program for you that includes yoga.

What Yoga Is *Not*

First of all, yoga is not a sport. Nor is it a religion. Did we hear a big sigh of relief? Good.

If you're not an athlete, you might find it quite appealing that yoga isn't competitive. A sense of competitiveness is in direct opposition to the yogi's frame of mind. Your yoga practice is individual and unique to you.

In yoga, it doesn't matter whether you approach it for fitness, stress relief, enlightenment, or healing. It doesn't matter how physically advanced you are, whether you are out of shape and inflexible or an athlete extraordinaire. If you practice yoga, it will help you in whatever way you require.

Though you may choose to blend a spiritual mind-set into yoga, it's certainly not required. Yoga in and of itself is not a religion, though it can complement and enhance spiritual development. The ideas and nonviolent philosophies in yoga can enhance any belief system.

The key to getting the most benefit out of yoga is to be clear about setting your intention before you begin. What do you want to get out of your yoga practice? You don't need to begin

dhyana, a daily meditation practice, to find your answer. The answer can be simple: it's up to you.

> **Know Your Sanskrit** _____
> Dhyana *(dee-YAH-nah)* means meditation—the process of quieting the mind to free yourself from preconceptions and illusions. The result is a clearer vision of the truth about yourself, your life, and the world.

Set Your Mind Free

People have been practicing yoga for thousands of years, not because they want to be "in shape" (a fringe benefit), but because they seek meaning in life. Yoga can be a fitness program, but it can also be a path to greater self-knowledge and, ultimately, self-actualization. Yoga helps you reach the fullness of your human potential. You will be more confident, stronger, healthier, and more at peace with who you are. You will make better decisions, set and achieve worthwhile goals, and become the person you want to be.

The ultimate goal of the yogi is to achieve the experience of truth, which might mean different things to different people, but which is, to some degree, a consistent experience for all—a clarity of vision, supreme focus, and a feeling of oneness with the profound nature of things, even the universe. This ideal state is called *samadhi* and involves consciousness to such a heightened degree that individual ego falls away and oneness with the universal force of love and goodness, or *brahman*, is achieved. It is the state of pure bliss.

But wait a minute! Didn't we just say this wasn't a religion? Again, it's up to you to create your personal definition of brahman, whether it be God, Goddess, Creator, Jesus, Allah, Buddha, Divine Being, Nature, Full Consciousness, or Higher Power. You decide how you will form the intentions of your yoga practice.

Know Your Sanskrit

Samadhi *(sah-MAH-dee)* is the goal of yoga. It's when the yogi finally becomes aware of nothing but brahman *(BRAH-mahn)*—the all-pervading Supreme Self, or God—everywhere. It's a state of absolute bliss and might be transitory or, ideally, perpetual.

Samadhi can be an elusive experience in our high-paced world. On the other hand, it's quite easy to get occasional glimpses or sudden rushes of bliss that fall away but become imprinted in our memories. Your world is what you make it, and yoga can help you optimize yourself, your experiences, and your all-important perception of the world around you. Yoga is fitness plus peace and fitness plus joy.

Your Body and Yoga

Yoga can help you optimize the particular physical body you've been given, but your physical makeup isn't the whole picture. You are also animated by energy. Your cultural background determines the way you see or understand your body in all its layers and complexities, and your own personal level of confidence and trust in your own body can teach you even more about the complex package otherwise known as you. Yoga can teach you to accept yourself on all levels. It can teach you to appreciate your body as it is now, and begin the journey to explore your bodymind and reach your true center.

Where Do You Stand?

To see how aware you are in your body right now, stand up, with your feet together, and lift your toes up from the floor. See if you can feel your arches slightly rise as you do this. If you can feel this, try to maintain the lift of the arches as you lower your toes. Also notice whether your hips are square. Is your weight evenly distributed? Notice how you hold your shoulders. Are they slumped? Are they up around your ears? Good posture increases the flow of prana through your body. Yoga will teach you how to maintain good posture.

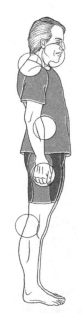

Poor posture blocks the flow of prana.

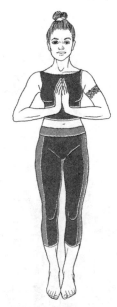

Prayer pose centers, restores, and renews. Inhale and lift your heart. Exhale and lower your shoulders.

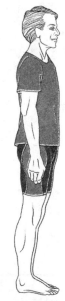

Yoga practice helps you align your body for increased energy and vitality.

Your Personal Energy Cycle

Let's face it, some of us are morning people, and some of us are night owls. Some of us are go-go-go types, and others are slow-slow-slow. Then, again, most of us experience a little of both. Our energy fluctuates. Various factors are at work: increased physical activity, too little sleep, overeating, menstrual cycles for women, the weather.

A Yoga Minute

Are you a night owl or a lark? Typical larks enjoy the morning and a good breakfast, feel most alert and creative early in the day, and prefer to retire early. Night owls often dislike eating breakfast, enjoy their peak later in the day, and prefer to stay up late and sleep in.

A regular yoga practice will smooth out your natural energy flow. When energy shoots up or plummets too suddenly, you are left feeling exhausted and out of balance. Instead of super highs and abysmal lows, you can enjoy a steady stream of energy. With the regular practice of yoga, your energy levels instead of shifting abruptly will blend more easily.

Yoga helps you get in touch with and pay closer attention to these cycles as it softens the transitions between them. Your natural energy flow is enhanced, which makes your daily movements easier and more enjoyable.

The Muscle and Bone Connection

Yoga postures demonstrate a great understanding of how your bones and muscles work together. Your skeleton contains 206 bones and supports your muscles and organs. Connecting the muscles to the bones are tendons. Muscles help you bend your joints and perform all sorts of tasks. Strong muscles go a long way toward supporting your frame, making it easier to achieve good posture.

Yoga is the caretaker of the spine, lengthening and extending it to release the energy that runs through this neural superhighway. The *chakras* are energy centers that are aligned on the spine, rising from the base to the crown. The chakras take in and release prana.

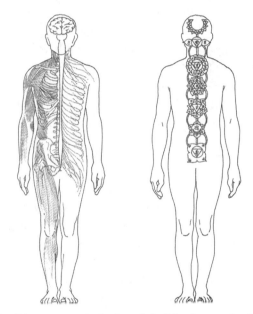

The Western anatomical model of the human body's musculoskeletal and nervous systems (left) is complemented by yoga's seven energy centers, called chakras (right), which store and release prana, the life force.

Know Your Sanskrit

Chakras (*CHAH-krahs*) are centers of energy located between the base of your spinal column and the crown of your head. Each chakra has a corresponding color, sound, perception, and biological function. Note that the actual spelling of chakra is cakra, but this spelling isn't commonly used. For more about chakras, see Appendix B.

Mind Meet Body, Body Meet Mind

Beginning to practice yoga is like introducing your body and your mind for the first time. In yoga, the body, mind, and spirit are closely intertwined. Hatha Yoga is the perfect introduction to this synergy because it concentrates on strengthening and purifying the physical body while simultaneously strengthening and purifying the mind. Practicing Hatha Yoga means finding the balance in the union of your bodymindspirit. Hatha Yoga is truly a holistic exercise.

The Western approach to yoga tends to be more fitness-oriented, while the Eastern approach to yoga is based on the idea that a healthy body makes it easier to progress spiritually. Either approach benefits both body and mind, however. If you're interested in yoga for its physical benefits, you can consider the spiritual centeredness you achieve a splendid bonus. Or if you tend more toward the Eastern way, consider fitness the icing on the cake. Either way, yoga fitness power means self-confidence, self-control, and inner peace. Whatever your fitness level, let yoga challenge you.

Coming Back to Center

Focusing on your breath and clearing your mind at the beginning of a yoga session are vital. The breath brings you back to mindfulness. The mindfulness anchors you in your body and the present moment. You'll notice you can concentrate better on the poses. You'll notice that you can find your center of gravity more easily. Start each session by setting your intention, whether it be for tranquility, wholeness, or confidence.

You may have heard the term "centering," and wondered what in the world this means. Centering means that you draw your breath and life force energy within, releasing all distractions. You find the calmness you carry within but sometimes lose sight of when you are concerned about the world around you. Many people find it helps to start a yoga session by closing their eyes and drawing in deep breaths until the busy mind quiets.

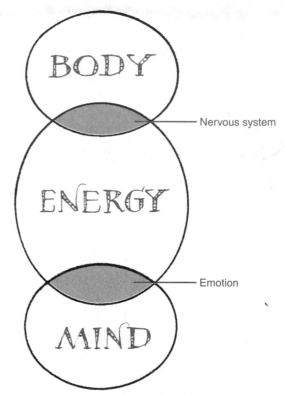

Pure energy transcends mind and body. Our emotions and nervous systems are physical links to energy. Pure energy transcends the physical.

It's All in Your Mind!

Whether you are an athlete or a ballet dancer, a bravo performance hinges on the right frame of mind. There is a point at which maximum performance can be achieved, when the performer is in the flow-state. Suddenly, your skill is heightened, your mind is sharp, and you can do no wrong. When you are "in the zone," your performance becomes flawless, and you're able to exceed your normal abilities.

Yoga is like a key to the secret door into the zone. Because yoga unites body and mind, it teaches you to discipline your mental state just as it teaches you discipline over your muscles. Your mind can be the instrument that keeps you in the zone of peak performance. Yoga unlocks the secret door to new productivity, creativity, efficiency, and true delight.

Wise Yogi Tells Us

End every yoga session with a few minutes of complete and total relaxation. Don't move, don't think; practice sitting or lying absolutely still. Simply feel your body. This little space at the end of your yoga workout is an important part of bringing your mind and body together—grounding your awareness and allowing your body to make the most of your workout.

Carry It Forward

The benefits of a yoga session can spill over into the rest of your life. Do you have a big presentation at work? You are calm, confident, and empowered. Do you have a championship tennis match? You are strong, flexible, buoyant, and the ball seems to go exactly where you will it to go. Do you have a really difficult test? Your mind is so uncluttered that all your studying comes back to you effortlessly.

Of course, success doesn't necessarily come overnight. Yoga is a process. Your bodymind needs to learn new habits and new modes of intercommunication. But if you're persistent and follow the yoga path, you'll quickly perceive the changes blessing your life. You'll more often feel your mind at peace, even perhaps the ecstasy of oneness with the life force. And you will be in the best shape you've ever been, too. So what are you waiting for?

The Least You Need to Know

- ◆ Yoga is a full-body workout that enhances the mind and spirit, too.
- ◆ Hatha Yoga is the most commonly practiced branch of yoga in the West. It emphasizes the physical.
- ◆ Yoga is user friendly. It's easy to get started, and it's easy on your body.
- ◆ In yoga, body, mind, and spirit are closely intertwined.

In This Chapter

- ◆ The history of yoga
- ◆ The nine types of yoga
- ◆ Yoga dos and don'ts
- ◆ Yoga and spirituality

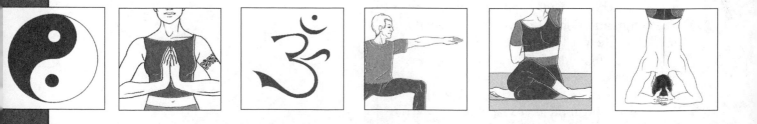

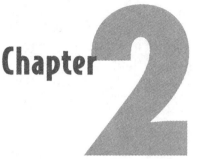

Chapter 2

Yoga's Spiritual Tradition

It's true that you don't have to know anything about the yoga tradition to practice yoga. But yoga has an illustrious and ancient history, and understanding its deep and sagacious roots might help you gain a deeper appreciation of yoga's staying power. Blending yoga's guidelines for living into your practice will almost certainly enrich your life.

In this chapter, we will explore the sacred origins of yoga and identify the many styles of yoga. Along the way, we'll introduce you to some of the sacred ancient texts and yoga's central values.

The Origin of Yoga

Yoga has been around for a long, long time. "How long?" you ask. Well, elements of yoga are in the *Rig Veda*, possibly the oldest known text in the world, which goes back 4,000 years. Because little written text exists, no one knows for sure the exact origin of yoga, though yoga exercises are included in texts of ayurveda, an ancient Indian system of health.

One of the best known texts on yoga is Patanjali's Eightfold Path, which was written several thousand years before Christ. It's a collection of pithy, sometimes enigmatic aphorisms that describe yoga's purpose, practice, and guidelines for living. Patanjali's Eightfold Path is still used today as the quintessential yoga reference.

But for most of us, our first awareness of yoga likely has its origin in the burgeoning interest in the 1960s in all things Eastern. The rock group The Beatles befriended Maharishi Mahesh Yogi and incorporated Hindu melodies in songs such as "Norwegian Wood (This Bird Has Flown)" and "Within You Without You." It was a time when traditional values were being questioned and yoga offered an alternative set of values attractive to spiritual seekers.

Today, yoga is more popular than ever before. We are seeking the spiritual with new vigor as an answer to a world we can't control—and not just the spiritual in theory. We are seeking the spiritual in *action*, in a way that can be meaningful to each of us. The way yoga has taken hold thousands of years later in Western culture illustrates just how timeless it is.

A Yoga Minute

Maharishi Mahesh Yogi was the inventor of Transcendental Meditation, or TM, a form of meditation that uses the ancient concept of mantra or repetition of sacred sounds.

Because yoga encourages the study of the sacred (*svadhyaya*), you might find it interesting, even helpful, to take a look at some of the world's major spiritual texts. Reading and studying any or even all of them will benefit your yoga practice as well as expand your mind to new possibilities.

Here are a few of the major sacred texts of India:

- The **Rig Veda,** considered the most ancient of sacred texts. Meaning "Knowledge of Praise," it's been orally passed down via Hindu priests who were trained to memorize the hymns precisely. Consisting of 1,028 hymns, the *Rig Veda* is now believed to be more than 4,000 years old.

- The **Upanishads,** the scriptures of ancient Hindu philosophy, which describe the path of Jnana Yoga, the discipline of wisdom as a path to self-realization.

- The **Bhagavad Gita** is one of India's most beloved and famous sacred texts. It tells the epic story of the warrior-prince Arjuna as he stands at the edge of a battlefield preparing for war. He discusses his universal moral dilemmas with the Hindu god Krishna, who is driving Arjuna's chariot. Is war justified? What if your loved ones are on the opposing side? What is right when your duties conflict? What does it mean to be born, to live, to die? It's a beautiful story of inner quests and spiritual awakenings.

- Patanjali's **Yoga Sutras,** the source of Patanjali's Eightfold Path. Many call Patanjali the father of yoga because of this significant and influential text, but the practice of yoga was around long before Patanjali's text.

- The **Hatha-Yoga-Pradipika,** a fourteenth-century guide to Hatha Yoga—everything you always wanted to know about Hatha Yoga but were afraid to ask!

Planting the Seeds: Yoga Branches for All Growing Personalities

Our focus in this book is on Hatha Yoga, but there are many different branches of yoga, each with its own distinctive path. Though each branch emphasizes a different path, the goal is unified: a state of pure bliss and oneness with the universe. Here's a closer look at these yoga branches, which are summarized in a table at the end of this list:

- **Hatha Yoga: Know your body, know your mind.** As we've mentioned before, Hatha Yoga works under the assumption that supreme control over the body, or the physical self, is one path to enlightenment. Hatha Yoga is a sort of spiritual fitness plan in which balance is key. Attention to the physical is foremost in Hatha Yoga;

this particular type of yoga involves cleansing rituals and breathing exercises designed to manipulate the body's energy through breath control and body positioning.

> **Wise Yogi Tells Us** _____
>
> If you're ill, whether you have a cold, chronic pain, or something more serious, start slow, as little as five minutes a day. Even taking a series of full, deep breaths can be centering to body and mind.

◆ **Raja Yoga: Know your mind, know the universe.** Raja Yoga, also known as *The Royal Path*, emphasizes control of the intellect to attain enlightenment. Meditation, concentration, and breath control are paramount in Raja Yoga. Hatha Yoga is sometimes considered a stepping-stone to Raja Yoga, because after control of the body is mastered, control of the mind comes more easily.

◆ **Kriya Yoga: Put it in action.** Kriya means "spiritual action." The practice of Kriya Yoga involves quieting the mind through scriptural self-study, breathing techniques, mantras, and meditation. Kriya Yoga understands that divine energy is stored in the lower part of the body. Like Kundalini Yoga, Kriya Yoga breathing and meditation techniques help bring this energy up the spine.

> **Wise Yogi Tells Us** _____
>
> The differences between the schools of yoga can be subtle or they can appear quite significant. Keep in mind that when it all comes down to it, yoga is about uniting, not differentiating. In the end, it's all yoga!

◆ **Karma Yoga: Put it into service.** Karma Yoga emphasizes selfless action. The follower of Karma Yoga proceeds through daily life attempting to increase virtue and decrease lawlessness in the world by working for others and foregoing personal desires, resulting in greater empathy for and understanding of the world—and eventually, full understanding, or enlightenment.

Karma is the law of cause and effect, or "what goes around comes around." Everything you do, say, or think has an immediate effect in the universe and in you. Karma is not negative. It is neither bad nor good. It is the movement toward balanced consciousness.

◆ **Bhakti Yoga: Open your heart.** Bhakti Yoga places sincere, heartfelt devotion to the divine ahead of all else. Bhakti Yoga involves reverence, devotion, and perpetual remembrance of whatever divine presence is meaningful to you. Bhakti Yoga's focus is the heart, and the development of compassion is cultivated as the primary way to achieve unity with the divine.

◆ **Jnana Yoga: Sagacious you.** Jnana Yoga is the path of knowledge and wisdom. Inquiring minds are what Jnana Yoga is all about, and because all knowledge is hidden within us, Jnana Yoga's goal is to inquire deeply into ourselves through questioning, meditation, and contemplation until we find that knowledge. Jnana Yoga involves a radical shift in perception. The intellect, or the mind, is given the major workout focus in Jnana Yoga.

Type of Yoga	The Path	Emphasis	Methods
Hatha	Supreme control of body	The body	Poses, or asanas Breathing exercises Cleansing rituals
Raja	Enlightenment of the mind	Discipline of intellect	Meditation Concentration Breath control
Kriya	Spiritual action	Releasing divine energy up the spine	Spiritual self-study Breathing techniques Mantras
Karma	Service	Selfless action	Increase virtue in daily life Work for others Forego personal desires Cultivate empathy
Bhakti	Unity with divine	Devotion	Reverance Remembrance Love
Jnana	Knowledge and wisdom	Self-discovery	Self-inquiry Meditation Contemplation Shift in perception
Tantra	Using ritual to achieve enlightenment	Ritual, channeling energy, weaving your energy with divine energy	Study of sacred writings and physical rituals
Mantra	Using sound to expand enlightenment	Sounds that affect consciousness	Singing Chanting Rhythm Recitation
Kundalini	Awakening energy	Achieving balance between compassion and awakening	Energy channels charged Breathwork Movement

◆ **Tantra Yoga: Rituals and you.** The common misconception in the West is that Tantra Yoga is about sexual rituals. But Tantra is a complex, ancient, and esoteric discipline involving sacred rituals based on the idea that humans are a reflection of divinity. Tantra Yoga involves the techniques of ritual and study to channel energy, reveal the divine, and achieve enlightenment. The word *tantra* means "weaving" and it is through ritual that one "weaves" oneself with the divine and achieves enlightenment.

Tantra *does* recognize the power of sexual energy, and for that reason it has become most famous in Western culture for the notion that sexual energy is an important store of energy that can be rechanneled to further spiritual enlightenment.

◆ **Mantra Yoga: The sound of enlightenment.** Mantra Yoga is the study of sacred sounds. A mantra is a syllable or sequence of syllables designed to clear the mind and encourage spiritual awakening. We'll talk about mantras in Chapter 9.

Mantra Yoga centers on the principle that sound can affect consciousness. *Aum* (often spelled *Om*) is the most commonly known mantra syllable and sounds curiously (but probably not coincidentally) like "amen," the sound that punctuates so many religious hymns and prayers.

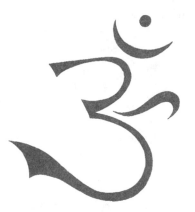

Aum, written in Sanskrit.

◆ **Kundalini Yoga: Awakening.** Kundalini Yoga is the study of kundalini (energy) movement along the spine, which is released—awakened—through breath and specific Hatha Yoga movements. Kundalini Yoga involves techniques meant to awaken energy, which is symbolized as a snake that "sleeps" at the base of the spine. When released correctly (that is, when the recipient is properly prepared), kundalini energy, sometimes called "serpent power," is potent and results in enlightenment. If released too soon, kundalini energy mixes with a person's negative emotions and can turn into intense and painful experiences. Pure kundalini is a balanced and compassionate source of energy.

Yoga's Rules to Live By

If you're the kind of person who likes a nice, clean set of rules to live by, Patanjali's guidelines are for you. In his *Yoga Sutras*, he outlined yoga's Eightfold Path. Even today, these guidelines can offer a structure for your yoga practice and your daily life. Here's a quick version of the Eightfold Path:

1. Yoga don'ts (yamas):

   Nonviolence (ahimsa)

   Nonlying (satya)

   Nonstealing (asteya)

   Nonpursuit of lust/desire (brahmacharya)

   Nongreed (aparigraha)

2. Yoga do's (niyamas):

   Purity (saucha)

   Contentment (santosha)

   Self-discipline (tapas)

   Self-study (svadhyaya)

   Devotion (ishvar-pranidhana)

3. Yoga poses (asanas)

4. Breathing exercises (pranayama)

5. Detachment (pratyahara)

6. Concentration (dharana)

7. Meditation (dhyana)

8. Pure consciousness (samadhi)

Yoga Don'ts: Just Say No (Yamas)

The "don'ts" of yoga aren't meant to keep you bound by restrictions, but rather to help you grow by purifying your body and your mind. Practicing them can teach you self-discipline. You might also find that you already live by many of them.

Yamas (*YAH-mahs*) are five abstinences or forms of discipline that purify the body and mind: ahimsa (*ah-HIM-sah*) means nonviolence, satya (*SAHT-ya*) means truthfulness, asteya (*ah-STAY-yah*) means nonstealing, brahmacharya (*BRAH-mah-CHAR-yah*) means chastity or nonlust, and aparigraha (*ah-PAH-ree-GRAH-hah*) means nongreed.

◆ **Do no harm (ahimsa).** Ahimsa comprises your actions, words, and thoughts. The highest level is to refrain from violent thoughts. Wish your enemies well, and your heart will lighten. According to yoga, we are all energy, and our thoughts can be sensed on the energetic level, so our thoughts do go out into the world. It is better to transform your negative thoughts than to hide them. Yoga provides a method for doing this. (And remember this applies to your own self-talk, too!)

A Yoga Minute

According to the Institute of Science, Technology, and Public Policy, more than 40 studies have demonstrated that large groups practicing organized meditation (specifically, Transcendental Meditation in these studies) in one location reduce social stress and violence in urban, metropolitan, and even national areas. For more information on specific studies about meditation and reduced violence, see www.kosovopeace.org/research.html.

◆ **Tell no lies (satya).** The second yama involves truthfulness. But what is the truth? You and I have different truths, so isn't truth changeable? According to yoga philosophy, truthfulness is the result of our mind, speech, and actions being unified and harmonious. Truth does no harm and results in personal integrity and strength of character.

◆ **Do not steal (asteya).** Maybe you would never think of shoplifting, but have you ever taken credit for someone else's ideas? This concept extends to not interrupting people, because that steals their thunder. Another example would be not purchasing products stolen by others. Every choice you make resonates all over the world, even into future generations. We have more personal power than we think when it comes to correcting injustice, locally and globally. Yoga can help us become aware of the power that comes from practicing asteya in all levels of our lives.

◆ **Cool it, Casanova (brahmacharya).** Brahmacharya is about virtue, but it doesn't mean you'll never have sex again. (Did we hear a sigh of relief?) Brahma means "truth," and *char* means "to move," so brahmacharya essentially means "to control the movement of truth." Lust and desire, in their many forms, obscure truth. Developing the inner strength to control our lusts and desires helps us see truth more clearly. In other words, brahmacharya is a movement toward responsible behavior and a higher truth beyond the physical.

◆ **Don't be greedy (aparigraha).** Aparigraha means living simply, possessing only what is necessary, and recognizing that possessions are merely tools to use in life. Accumulations, whether material things or unnecessary thoughts, tie you down to this world. Simplify your life as you simplify your thoughts.

Greed can also surface in less obvious ways. Talking too much, interrupting others, and dominating conversations while barely showing a flicker of interest in the participation of others are all ways greed creeps into our lives through language.

Yoga Do's: Just Say Yes (Niyamas)

And now for the fun part! *Niyamas* are Patanjali's observances—what to do, as opposed to what *not* to do. The first niyama cleanses the way for all the others.

Niyamas are observances or personal disciplines. There are five: saucha (*SAH-chah*) means purity or inner and outer cleanliness, santosha (*san-TOH-shah*) means contentment, tapas (*TAH-pahs*) means self-discipline, svadhyaya (*svahd-YAH-yah*) means self-study, and ishvara-pranidhana (*ISH-var-ah PRAH-nee-DAH-nah*) means centering on the divine.

- **Be pure (saucha).** You achieve purity through the practice of the five previous yamas, so the yamas and niyamas work hand in hand. The abstentions clear away negative physical and mental states of being, leading you straight to purity.

  Purity can apply to various aspects of your life—cleanliness, neatness, and healthful eating. Many yogis are vegetarians because they believe they should only eat food obtained through purer, nonviolent means.

- **Be content (santosha).** Just saying the word santosha produces a sense of calm. Practicing contentment means finding happiness with what you have and with who you are. Contentment helps you see that you're exactly where you're supposed to be right now.

  Contentment means learning to reevaluate obstacles as opportunities. Practicing contentment involves taking full responsibility for your life and the situations you're in. No blame games are necessary. You're in the driver's seat!

> **Wise Yogi Tells Us**
>
> Feeling discontented? Try this exercise. Create a list of everything that makes you discontented. Then rewrite your list, finding a way to see each source of discontentment in some positive light. For example, rewrite "I hate my job" to "My job has taught me that I am more creative than I thought." When you're finished, throw away that first list—you don't need it!

- **Be disciplined (tapas).** For all the yamas and niyamas to be truly effective, you'll need self-discipline. Not your strong point? Learning how to stick to something even when you don't feel like it builds your strength, wisdom, and sense of empowerment. The yamas and niyamas themselves provide an excellent opportunity to practice self-discipline.

  Self-discipline is difficult for almost everyone, but changing your attitude might help keep you on track. The best way to do this is to focus on the positive: "I will relax with deep-breathing exercises tonight." "I will have a soothing cup of herbal tea this morning." Focusing on the positive makes being disciplined more fun. Because really, discipline isn't deprivation, it's self-care.

- **Be studious (*svadhyaya*).** Svadhyaya means studying yourself through introspection. The word means "inquiring into your own nature, the nature of your beliefs, and the nature of the world's spiritual journey." You accomplish this by studying sacred texts such as the *Bhagavad Gita* or the Bible. Through self-study, you can see which thoughts, actions, words, and experiences bring you closer to the core of who you really are.

◆ **Be devoted (ishvara-pranidhana).** The last niyama involves devotion. Focusing on the divine is represented differently for different people. This yama often misleads people into thinking that yoga is a religion. Some people might perceive it this way, but this yama is simply a call to move closer to the essence of who you are. Nurturing your spirituality is an important part of balancing your whole self, which is yoga's realm.

Yoga's Other Pathways

The rest of the Eightfold Path provides some of the basic techniques for yoga practice:

◆ **Body control (asana).** Body control, or asana, is both an important part of yoga and its most well-known component. Remember that body control is not the only path, but merely one path yoga offers. Asana literally translates as "posture" and is derived from the Sanskrit root *as*, which means "to stay."

◆ **Breath control (pranayama).** Prana refers to the life force or energy that exists everywhere and is manifested in each of us through the breath. Ayama means "to stretch or extend." Prana flows out from the body, and pranayama teaches us to maneuver and direct prana for optimal physical and mental benefit.

◆ **Detachment (pratyahara).** Pratyahara is the practice of withdrawing the senses from everything that stimulates them. Normally, we live by our senses. We listen, we look, we taste, we touch, and we smell. This is the ordinary state of things, but it's also a state we can temporarily suspend in favor of a deeper awareness.

Ouch!

Are you feeling listless, depressed, and under the weather? According to ancient yoga texts, you have too much prana outside your body. Prana is constantly moving and flowing into and out of us, and pranayama is a tool for maintaining your health and well-being. Keep yourself healthier and happier by using breath control to keep more prana inside (where it belongs)!

◆ **Concentration (dharana).** *Dhri* means to hold. Dharana involves concentration—to hold your mind on a single point. The practice of dharana involves teaching the mind to hold one thing instead of many. Dharana works hand in hand with meditation. The goal is to become aware of nothing but the object on which you are concentrating, whether it's a candle flame, a flower, or a mantra. The purpose is to train the mind to gently push away superfluous thought.

◆ **Meditation (dhyana).** Dhyana, or meditation, can be defined as being linked to the object of your concentration so that nothing else exists. It's keen, heightened awareness, not nothingness. Your mind is completely focused and quiet yet awake and very aware.

◆ **Pure consciousness (samadhi).** All the limbs of yoga lead to samadhi, the final limb of the Eightfold Path. Samadhi means to merge, and this state of pure consciousness means just that: a complete and total merging with the object of your meditation. When in a state of samadhi, you understand not only that you and the object of your meditation are one, but that you and the universe are one. Samadhi is pure, total bliss.

Yoga Embraces All

So with such a rich history and belief system, you might suspect that yoga must surely be a religion. Yoga does offer guidelines for living, encourage study of sacred texts, and facilitate communion with the "divine." Some branches of yoga seem more religious or mystical than others, but yoga itself is certainly *not* a religion.

Yoga is open to all religions. Yoga is not biased, prejudiced, or exclusive. You needn't be a Hindu, a Buddhist, a Muslim, a Christian, or a Jew. Whether you are religious or not, yoga will help you understand your beliefs more clearly and get you in closer touch with your spiritual nature.

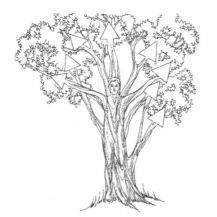

Growing with Yoga's Eightfold Path.

The Least You Need to Know

◆ Different types of yoga—Hatha, Raja, Kriya, Karma, Bhakti, Jnana, Tantra, Mantra, and Kundalini—emphasize different practices but have the same goal: enlightenment.

◆ You don't have to be spiritual to practice yoga, but if you practice yoga, you'll probably end up being a little more spiritual.

◆ Yoga offers guidelines for living.

◆ The five abstentions are nonviolence, non-lying, nonstealing, nonlusting, and non-greed.

◆ The five observances are purity, contentment, self-discipline, self-study, and devotion.

◆ Yoga also involves body control, breath control, detachment, concentration, and meditation.

In This Chapter

- ◆ The foundation poses of Hatha Yoga
- ◆ Linking it together
- ◆ Balancing opposing forces
- ◆ Integrating all aspects of you

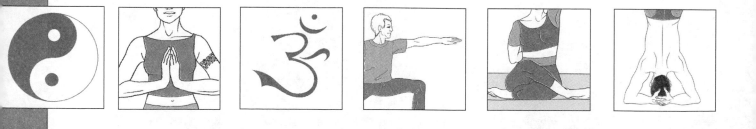

Hatha Yoga Basics

Hatha Yoga is more than a classic yoga path—it's the path of self-mastery. The asanas, or the poses, of Hatha Yoga are the heart of its practice, and they point the way to full integration of self. Breath and meditation play a strong role, and are also essential components of Hatha's physical execution of the poses.

In our physically oriented culture, it comes as no surprise that Hatha Yoga is by far the most common yoga practice in the West. Despite that, it's clear that the surge of interest in yoga is driven by people discovering there's more to yoga than stretching and breathing.

Strike a Pose

Hatha Yoga's power lies in physical discipline. In Hatha Yoga, you train your body to move into specific positions and hold them, using the breath to enhance the pose. Eventually, even difficult poses become exercises in meditation. The poses of Hatha Yoga are by no means random. They are specifically designed to activate the internal as well as the external aspects of the body. Hatha Yoga introduces us to our personal realm of physical possibilities.

In this chapter, we will introduce you to the basic Hatha Yoga poses.

Standing Poses

Mountain pose, or tadasana, forms the foundation for the standing poses. Standing poses develop and strengthen your legs. Standing poses also improve your balance, align your hips and spine, and maintain equilibrium throughout your body. Master the standing poses before you attempt the more complicated ones, such as balance poses and floor poses that require more advanced flexibility and/or strength. If you practice standing poses regularly, you'll notice an almost immediate improvement in your leg and hip flexibility, as well as increased strength and general stability throughout your entire body. Your balance and posture will improve, too.

Okay, you say, I stand all the time. I don't need to practice that. You might be tempted to flip ahead and find a pose that is more challenging, but we urge you to take a closer look. In perfecting Mountain pose, you set yourself up for practicing more difficult poses with grace and ease. Mountain pose is the starting place from which all the other standing poses form.

Posture Perfect

Remember breathing into Prayer pose in Chapter 1? Good posture is essential to proper form in doing yoga's standing poses—and the seated ones, too. Proper posture looks better, feels better—and quite simply, *is* better for your body.

How can you work consciously to improve your posture? The discipline of Hatha Yoga's standing poses carries over into how you move in all aspects of life. Try it. During the day, whether you're in line at the grocery store or filling up at the gas station, notice *how* you're standing.

Wise Yogi Tells Us

Here's an easy way to maintain good posture while standing: pretend you have a loop attached to the crown of your head and a string tied to the loop. Imagine someone above you is pulling on the string. Feel how your entire spine and neck shift and stretch as the string pulls upward. That's what healthy posture feels like!

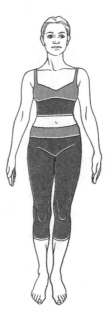

Mountain pose is Hatha Yoga's most basic standing pose and a core yoga pose that must be deeply studied before attempting more challenging poses.

Warrior Spirit

The warrior poses could just be our favorites.
They are popular because they are fun and
empowering. But don't let the word warrior
mislead you—this isn't about combat!

We tend to think of warriors as wearing
armor. But in yoga, the warrior represents the
strength of openness and the expansion of consciousness. It takes tremendous strength to live
a life of nonviolence, which is the path of the
yogi warrior.

Ouch!

Warrior? you might ask. What about
nonviolence? Don't get hung up on
the warrior idea. It's not about tensing up like you are going into battle. The
most effective warriors stay calm, clear-
headed, and agile. To achieve the readi-
ness of a warrior—without the fight-or-flight
feeling that freezes you up—concentrate on
lifting the internal center of your body.

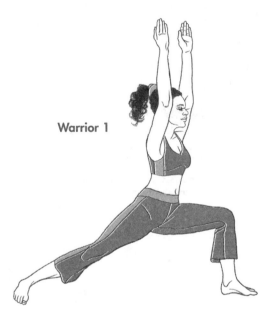

Warrior 1

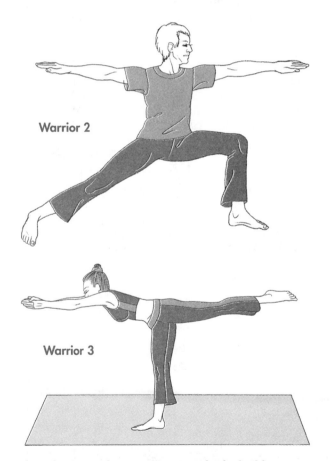

Warrior 2

Warrior 3

**The Warrior poses help strengthen body, mind, and spirit as they energize your body, build
confidence, improve balance, and provide strength.**

Forward Bends

Standing poses easily morph into forward bends. Forward bend poses can be standing or sitting poses. Forward bends stretch the back of the body and are essential for lengthening the muscles of the back, legs, shoulders, neck, and spine. Forward bends also activate many of the internal organ systems by compressing the organs as the front of your body folds over itself. That same folding inward can also help the mind focus inwardly for greater relaxation and a reflective, inner-gazing state. Learn standing poses and forward bends in Chapter 6.

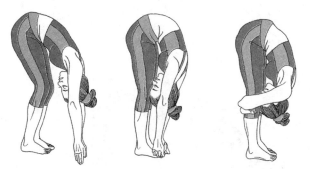

Standing Head to Knees pose lengthens the back of the body, helps stimulate internal organ function, and helps focus the mind on the inner self.

Backbends

Back-bending poses are the complements to forward-bending poses and balance each other in a yoga workout. Backbends stretch the front of the body, opening the chest, hips, and rib cage. They help to release emotions, open the heart, stretch and strengthen the muscles, and open the torso, releasing tension in the core body and the internal organs. We'll go into more depth on backbend poses in Chapter 7.

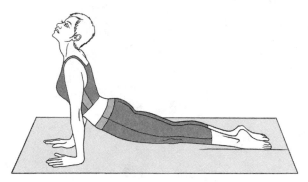

Upward Facing Dog is a basic back-bending pose that stretches the chest, strengthens the legs and arms, and helps open the heart for a freer flow of feeling.

Twists

We love twists, because they do amazing things for the spine. They open the joints of the hips and shoulders, add core flexibility, and can compress and stimulate internal organs in dramatic ways. Just be sure you always balance a twist by doing both sides. We'll go into spinal twists and more ways to move energy in your body in Chapter 8.

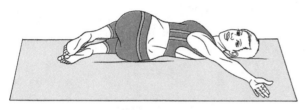

Basic twists like Lying Down Spinal Twist add flexibility to the spine and improve digestion and internal organ function.

Inversions

Inversions are lots of fun. Inversions give your body a break from its normal upright state and let you see the world upside down! Everything is turned topsy-turvy as your head goes down and your feet (depending on the pose) go up! Inversions help blood flow the opposite way in your body, flooding your brain and upper body with nourishment and giving your poor legs and feet a break from all that downward flow. Some people believe that a few minutes in an inverted pose every day can actually lengthen your life. We've personally tested this and sometimes we take a break from writing long enough to do a nice shoulder stand or headstand. Afterward, we feel refreshed and raring to go again, so the longevity merit certainly works for us in an "in the now" kind of way! Inversions are featured in Chapter 8.

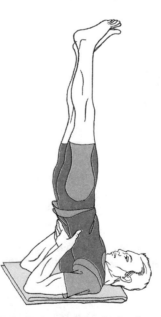

Shoulder Stand pose inverts the body, promoting blood flow to the head, neck, and shoulders, and directs fluids out of the feet and legs. Try it as a great mental refresher, not to mention a break for aching feet.

On the Floor

Time to move to the floor. Seated poses are an important part of yoga because they help you settle into a pose with less gravitational resistance. The primary poses are seated, meditative, and prone poses.

Seated Poses

Seated poses can involve many different kinds of poses, from easy to very challenging. Whether they involve a spinal twist, a hamstring stretch, or an abdominal strengthener, seated poses can benefit the body in a multitude of ways. Seated poses are featured in Chapter 9.

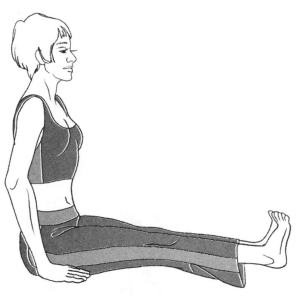

Staff pose is like Mountain pose for the floor. It encourages an inner strength and solidity, builds confidence, increases focus, and improves posture.

Meditative Poses

Meditative poses are just what they sound like: yoga poses suited for serious meditation. The most classic is the Lotus pose, but this challenging pose isn't for everybody, and beginners might want to wait and try it after they have more yoga experience. Other seated meditative poses might be more comfortable and more conducive to quiet contemplation. Once you've mastered Lotus, however, it is an ideal meditative pose for stability.

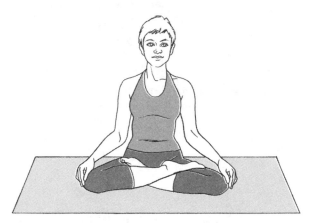

Lotus pose is the classic meditative yoga pose, designed to imitate the symmetry of the lotus flower and put the body in its most stable position for least distraction during meditation.

Prone Poses

Finally, prone poses are at the very heart of yoga, most particularly shavasana, or Corpse pose. This pose might look simple, but the deep meditative state it can help you achieve is what yoga is all about. Shavasana is a good way to end your yoga session. We'll take a closer look at shavasana in Chapter 12.

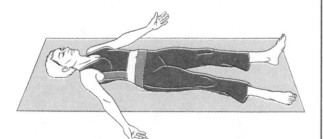

Shavasana, or Corpse pose, is a prone pose designed for deep and total bodymind relaxation.

 Wise Yogi Tells Us

Here's a common question Joan gets in her Yo Joan column:

Yo Joan: Why do we roll to the right side to come up from final relaxation pose?

Dear friend: The heart is on the left side of the body. Rolling to the right takes pressure off the heart.

Namaste,

Joan

You can find more "Yo Joan" questions and answers in Appendix A.

Vinyasana: One Thing Leads to Another

A vinyasana is a series of poses linked together in a dynamic sequence. Sun Salutation is an example of a yoga vinyasana. Practicing a vinyasana can be aerobically challenging and a lot of fun! Vinyasanas are used in Ashtanga Yoga, made popular by Sri K. Pattabhi Jois at the Ashtanga Yoga Research Institute in Mysore, India. This form of yoga links high-energy poses together in a sweat-inducing series of yoga challenges. Ashtanga Yoga is traditionally the yoga that specifically follows Patanjali's Eightfold Path as a way to enlightenment, but in the West we have come to associate the term with a highly athletic form of Hatha Yoga.

One version of ashtanga is power yoga. It's particularly popular in the fitness-conscious West, and has evolved into varying names according to the teacher and the teacher's teacher. Power yoga is a great introduction to yoga if you are highly athletic. Chapters 16, 17, and 18 offer ways to get started with *vinyasana* and other yoga sessions.

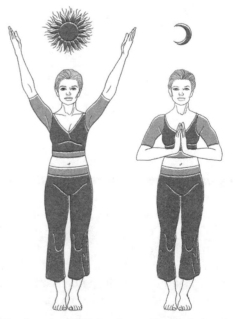

Yoga honors opposing forces that balance the human body within the powerful yet delicate balances of the universal body.

Joining the Sun and the Moon

Hatha Yoga is about balancing the opposing forces of the body, just as opposing forces are balanced outside the body. Sun and moon, male and female, day and night, cold and hot—the universe is made up of opposites.

The ancient Chinese symbol of yin and yang represents the idea of intermingling opposites. Notice that a white dot sits in the center of the fullest part of the black swirl, and vice versa. The symbol represents the concept that the dot of yang is the seed of yin, and the dot of yin is the seed of yang. One is always becoming the other.

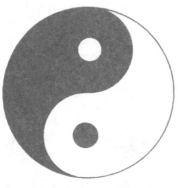

Yoga's yin/yang union.

Yin and yang are commonly associated with many different complementary qualities. Yin is primarily present in the moon, the night, cold, feminine energy, and heaviness. Yang is primarily present in the sun, the daytime, heat, masculine energy, and lightness. And because every force has an opposite and also contains a bit of its opposite within itself, masculine energy contains feminine energy, feminine energy contains masculine energy, night contains a bit of day, day contains a bit of night, and so on. So the universe goes—ultimately interconnected.

So goes your body, too. We are filled with opposites: a left and a right side, blood flowing to the heart and away from the heart, the delivery of nutrients and the removal of waste, inhalations and exhalations, hunger and satiety, sleeping and wakefulness, being with others and being alone, joy and sadness, birth and death, growth and decline. If any of the thousands of opposites and intricate balances within us become unbalanced, our bodies and minds won't work as efficiently.

Hatha Yoga balances us in many ways. Work on the left side is balanced with work on the right side. Forward-bending poses are followed by back-bending poses, contractions are followed by extensions, upright positions are followed by inversions, and so on. The practice of Hatha Yoga also balances our mental and spiritual energies, for what we do with the body affects the mind and the spirit (that triangle again!)—ultimately all are interconnected.

Balancing Prana

Yoga has a series of muscular exercises called *bandhas* that balance the movement of prana through the body. We draw prana into the body as we inhale. As we exhale, we generate energy, called *apana*, which moves away from the brain and carries impurities out of the body. Bandhas work like a fastener, binding good energy at points in the body to achieve a better state of balance.

Know Your Sanskrit

Bandha means to bind or to lock, and bandhas are muscular locks used during poses and breathing exercises to intensify the energy of prana and apana so it can eliminate impurities from the body. **Apana** is the energy generated in the body by exhalation that moves away from the brain and carries impurities out of the body.

The three primary bandhas are:

◆ **At the chin (jalandhara bandha).** When you bring your chin to your chest, you strengthen this bandha. It builds prana's upward movement.

◆ **In the abdominal solar plexus area (uddiyana bandha).** In any pose, when you pull your navel up and back toward your spine, you strengthen and build apana's movement down your spine.

◆ **In the area of the rectum (mula bandha).** When you contract your perineal muscle, you keep prana from escaping from your lower body. The perineal muscle is the muscle in front of the rectum. (For women: think Kegels!)

Bandhas are like checks and balances. They keep the system of balances in check by pulling everything toward a center point, intensifying the energy. Practicing these bandhas while sitting in meditation or holding a yoga pose can be a particularly powerful way of concentrating and intensifying *prana* in the body.

The result is that prana and apana are retained within the body, joining together within sushumna—the hollow passageway through your spinal cord. Their mingling generates an intense energy that can help awaken the kundalini serpent power. This joining of opposites, of prana and apana, of sun and moon, of ha and tha, is at the heart of Hatha Yoga's power.

Maybe you aren't too concerned with awakening your serpent power, especially because you aren't sure exactly what it is yet—or even whether you want to know. Maybe you are only vaguely aware of the importance of kundalini energy, but know that traditionally, this awakening of the "serpent power" is one of the primary purposes of Hatha Yoga.

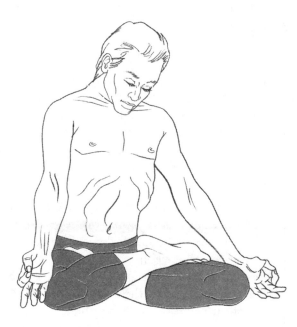

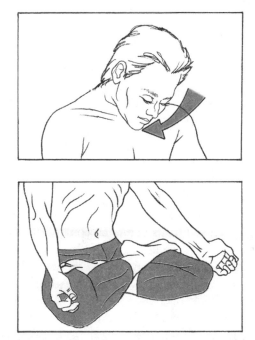

Practicing yoga's bandhas.

A Yoga Minute

In Hindu culture, the image of the kundalini serpent power doesn't have the negative connotation that serpents have in the West. In the Hindu religion, cobras are considered reincarnations of important people. Other cultures held the snake in reverence, too. The Aztecs worshipped a snake god who symbolized light, luck, and wisdom. In Africa, some cultures worship pythons, and killing snakes is a crime. Egyptian kings wore snake representations on their crowns, and the crosier of *Asklepios* (the Greek god of medicine and healing) is still a symbol of the medical profession today.

Physical fitness—making the body feel good and look good—has traditionally been a peripheral benefit, but it has shifted to the primary focus for Westerners. If fitness is your motivation for beginning Hatha Yoga practice, that's great. You'll benefit in many ways, no matter what reason brings you to the practice. But although fitness is important in Hatha Yoga, it means more than cut shoulders and washboard abs or lithe limbs and a toned tummy. Total fitness—of the mind, body, and spirit—is a far cry from body obsession. Body obsession is fitness gone awry.

Even if physical fitness is your primary goal, it doesn't hurt to be aware of the power of balanced opposites inherent in your practice. This heightened body awareness may move you to the more advanced paths of mental control (Raja Yoga) and spiritual awakening. Use Hatha Yoga to join the opposites of sun and moon within your body. Look back to the illustration earlier in this chapter of the greeting and honor to the sun from yoga's Sun Salutation vinyasana. The energies are drawn into the balanced, centered position of respect and thanks, *namaste*, or Prayer pose. You begin and end in a position of union and strength.

Know Your Sanskrit

Namaste (*nah-MAHS-tay*) means "Obeisance to you" or "I salute the divine light within you" and is a mudra (hand position) in which the palms and fingers come together in the prayer position. Your hands are held with your thumbs against your chest in an attitude of focused devotion. Namaste can also be held loosely behind your back with your fingers pointed up. Namaste is a greeting, symbolizing that as we go inward, we find there is no separation between us. Namascar refers to the act.

One Body ... or Three?

You have one body—or do you? Actually, according to yoga, you have three bodies: the physical body, the astral body, and the causal body. If the word "body" creates such a mental conundrum that you cannot imagine anything beyond the physical body, then it might be useful to think of these three bodies as energy fields—but it's energy that takes the form of *you*.

As you practice yoga, it is helpful to maintain an awareness of all three bodies. It will help you see more clearly the whole picture of you—to see how these energy fields work together to create the you that you know. Getting the full picture will help you see more clearly who you really are.

Within each of the bodies, or energy fields, exists five sheaths, or *koshas* (*KOH-shahs*), that make up the real you. Kosha is a Sanskrit word that means to envelope. The koshas, or envelopes, that make up the body are the physical body, the vital body, the mind sheath, the intellect sheath, and the sheath of bliss.

◆ The physical body is the crudest of the bodies and the smallest. This is the you in the mirror. Yet even though it's crude, it's your best tool for growth. You can't deny you have a physical body, so yoga helps you make the most of it. The first three aspects of Patanjali's Eightfold Path strengthen and train the physical body: abstinences (yamas), observances (niyamas), and poses (asanas).

◆ The vital body is a sheath within the physical body, where prana lives and moves. It often extends just beyond the physical body. Think of prana as the life force energy of the universe embracing you, and then you have the picture of the vital body.

◆ The astral body is the vehicle of the spirit and corresponds with the mind. This layer exists within the other two layers—the physical body and the causal body, which we describe next. Think of it as a second layer to your physical body, extending beyond the physical body but not to the limits of the causal body. To strengthen the astral body, turn to the next three steps of the Eightfold Path: breathing exercises (pranayama), sense withdrawal (pratyahara), and concentration (dharana).

The astral body encompasses the mind sheath and the intellect sheath. This is where you become aware of your emotions. This is where you become aware that you exist apart from your emotions.

◆ The causal body is the largest, most widely reaching layer of you, starting with spirit. It's the subtlest body and holds the spirit as well as the other layers. This is where you started. Individuality (as we normally think of it) exists to a minimal degree in the causal body, which allows the spirit to shine and truth to be evident. To experience the causal body, turn to the final two limbs of the Eightfold Path: meditation (dhyana) and superconsciousness or bliss (samadhi).

The causal body is sometimes called the bliss sheath. It contains all the energy that links you with the universe.

Hatha Yoga works under the assumption that the inner you is the you worth working on, but to get to the inner you, you must gain discipline over the outer you—your body. Hatha Yoga brings your physical body in balance so it doesn't impede the other bodies—the astral and causal. Only then can the self-actualized, balanced you emerge in your full glory.

What It All Means

Ultimately, what Hatha Yoga is all about is integration. In the state of samadhi, the self, including the body, blends into the universal energy we are all part of. All that bodywork is really just a way to learn how to transcend your body!

Keep your body in great condition. Know your body. Know your mind. Know yourself. That's the Hatha way.

The Least You Need to Know

◆ The primary Hatha Yoga poses consist of standing, forward-bending, back-bending, twisting, seated, meditative, and prone poses.

◆ Standing poses such as Mountain pose are the foundation for good posture.

◆ When you link together a series of poses in a dynamic sequence, it's called a vinyasana.

◆ Hatha Yoga is a balance of opposing forces.

◆ Training and toning your body through Hatha Yoga practice is a way of integrating all facets of yourself—body, mind, and spirit.

◆ Your physical body is one of many energy fields that make up the total you. Yoga unites the physical, causal, and astral bodies so that you may transcend the mere physical and access the spiritual world.

In This Chapter

- ◆ Choosing a yoga class and finding the right teacher
- ◆ Setting up a yoga practice at home
- ◆ Yoga on your own: multimedia style
- ◆ Squeezing yoga into your busy day
- ◆ What every yoga practice should include

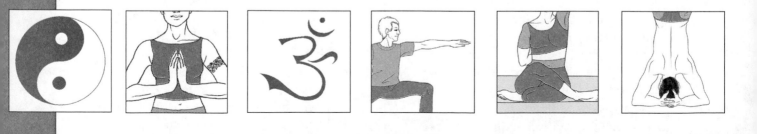

Chapter 4

Starting Your Yoga Practice

We know you'd like to just jump in and start with poses, but it's worth it to take a little extra time to make sure you set up the most favorable yoga experience for yourself. The ideal yoga routine is based on your personality, your schedule, your fitness level, your goals, and your learning style.

That said … it's time to make a yoga game plan. You may want to take a class and reap the benefits of a qualified instructor. Or you may want to try yoga on your own for a while; then consider a class later if you like the experience. In this chapter, we'll guide you in figuring out what to wear, what to buy, and when to squeeze it into your busy schedule.

Choosing a Yoga Class

Probably the best way to start out with yoga is to take a class. Real live instructors can best address your personal needs. During class, your instructor can see you from all angles, making minor adjustments in your poses to help you get the most benefit from each one. An instructor can also provide advice about the best postures for your particular physical challenges, such as a stiff neck, lower back pain, or tennis elbow. Plus, you'll learn from the other yoga practitioners in the class.

A regularly scheduled class will also keep you disciplined about your yoga practice. If you have to show up at a certain time, you might be less likely to put off or skip your practice.

Use the benefits of a qualified instructor and a regular class in conjunction with personal practice, and you'll really get up to speed quickly.

Yoga classes vary greatly in their format and approach, so if you do decide to take a class, you'll first want to do a bit of shopping. The right yoga class is highly personal.

Wise Yogi Tells Us _____

When you look for a yoga class, you have several factors to consider: the teacher's method and approach, the size of the class, class schedules, and location, to name a few. Plan on spending some time exploring the possibilities. It might take a while to find the right class and the right teacher for you, but many yogis believe that when the student is ready, the teacher will appear. Keep your mind and heart open.

Use our guide to yoga in Chapter 2 to help you select a teacher whose methods match your needs. But also talk to the teacher ahead of time to find out which school of yoga he or she practices and teaches to students. In addition to the branches of yoga described in Chapter 1, there are methods of teaching. Your instructor may teach a Hatha Yoga class, for instance, but be influenced by Iyengar.

Take into consideration some practicalities, such as the number of students in the class, the facilities, and the time. You'll want to make sure the class is small enough that the teacher can help you adjust your poses.

And by all means, if the first class doesn't feel right, don't give up—give feedback! Talk to your instructor. A different method may be better for you, and he or she may be able to recommend another yoga class you'll enjoy much more.

Wise Yogi Tells Us _____

Some good sources for finding a yoga class that suits your style are natural foods stores, health clubs or fitness centers, your health-care provider, or your local university or college.

Your Clothing: Keep It Loose

The right clothing is important, because if you can't move easily, if your clothes are in the way, or if you are in any way unnecessarily distracted (say, by a tight waist or stiff fabric), you won't be able to concentrate fully on your yoga poses.

There isn't any set yoga uniform, though yoga workout wear has gotten quite fashionable. You can choose to be fashionable or functional or both. But the most important guideline is to be comfortable.

You'll be most comfortable if your clothes are loose and flexible but not baggy. Tight clothes are restricting, and baggy clothes can get in the way of your movements. And if your clothes are baggy, it will be harder for you or your instructor to see if you are executing the poses correctly.

Also remember to dress properly for the temperature. If the room is cold, wear long sleeves and comfortable pants (sweatpants, leggings, or yoga pants). Many practitioners like to dress in layers, because you can heat up during some poses, but cool down during meditative poses.

Here are a few other tips to keep in mind:

◆ Yoga is best performed in bare feet. The more you practice yoga, the more sensitive and in tune with your environment you'll become, and that includes your feet!

◆ Don't forget to remove all metal jewelry before you practice, especially necklaces and bracelets. Yoga is about freeing the flow of energy in your body, and that energy could be disrupted by metal.

◆ Avoid wearing strong fragrances during your yoga practice. It can be unpleasant to others in your yoga class, especially during pranayama (breathwork), and some people are very sensitive to these smells.

An Equipment Commitment

But, you might wonder, how much should I invest in equipment if I am just trying out a class? It's a good idea to try a few classes before you shell out big bucks for that brightly colored yoga kit at the mall. All you really need to get started is your own body. Many yoga studios provide blankets and mats, when these are necessary.

The yoga kit you'll get at the mall may include a mat, a block, a belt, and a carrying case. The mat is useful for the floor poses, just to give you some cushioning and protect your clothing from dirt. The block you will use for balancing, and the belt will help you get the most out of a stretch.

Going Solo at Home

If you aren't quite ready for the commitment of a class, you'll find that it's quite easy to get set up at home. (And if you are taking a class, supplementing it with an at-home practice enhances the benefits you receive.) Do-it-yourself yoga can be very rewarding. You may use this book to design your own workout. All you need to do is find a comfortable place to practice and set a regular practice time.

Setting Up Your Practice Area

One of the great things about yoga is that you can do it almost anywhere—in the bedroom, in the living room, even outside! Your yoga place should definitely not be without these things, however:

- ◆ **A cushioned surface.** Nonskid carpets are good surfaces for practicing yoga, but if your floor isn't carpeted or is slippery, use a small nonskid rug or a sticky yoga mat.

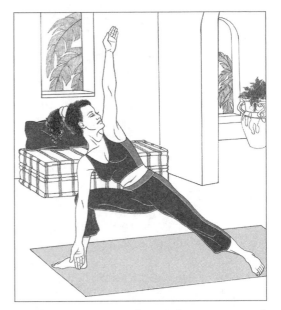

An at-home yoga space for regular practice can be a blissful sanctuary in your busy household.

- ◆ **A source of warmth.** Keep a blanket nearby to drape around yourself during still poses, breathing exercises, and meditation. Your muscles need to be warm to stay flexible. Practicing outside in the sun on a warm day is ideal. If you practice inside in the winter, consider a small electric heater for your practice area.

Ouch!

Keeping warm while practicing yoga is extremely important. If your muscles are cold, they can stiffen and lose flexibility, increasing your chance of injury. Warm muscles and joints are most conducive to a yoga workout. Also, in quieter poses and during meditation, you'll become colder more easily because you aren't encouraging active circulation.

◆ **Fresh air.** If you practice inside and weather permits, open a window and take a few deep breaths of fresh air before you start. Practicing outside—even better!

◆ **A clear area.** Practice in an area free of obstacles and distractions. Practicing yoga amid clutter and confusion is difficult and counterproductive.

Multimedia Yoga

Another great way to learn yoga is with a yoga video/DVD or audiotape/CD. One advantage of the audiotape/CD over the video/DVD is that you won't be glued to the television but can be directed inward instead.

A visit to your local library, video store, bookstore, or even the back pages of this very book will reveal a wealth of available audio and video references you can borrow, rent, or buy. A library or video store will permit you to sample a variety of yoga teachers and programs without committing. Once you've found a few you like, consider buying the CDs/DVDs for your personal collection. Then, whenever the desire strikes (2 A.M. on a Tuesday or 11 P.M. on a Friday), you can do yoga!

Yoga on the Net

The Internet is full of great yoga resources, from class schedules to "poses of the week" to peer support to spiritual guidance and inspiration. We list a few key websites in Appendix D, but one dearest to our hearts is YOYOGA!, if we do say so ourselves. Joan's website offers asanas of the week, yoga tips, massage tips, meditation tips, and other wonderful words of wonder, including the ever-popular "Yo Joan!" forum for all your yoga questions. Look up Joan at www.yoyoga.com.

When to Practice Yoga

It seems we're all stretched for time these days. But trust us, it's worth it to carve out time for a yoga routine. Your optimal yoga routine is the one that fits your lifestyle. You may want to start out with a once- or twice-a-week class, supplemented by sessions at home.

Ouch!

Though yoga isn't harsh to your body, it's important to give the body time between sessions to rest. Try practicing yoga for 20 minutes each morning on Mondays, Wednesdays, and Fridays. Or try it for 30 minutes after work and before dinner on Tuesdays and Thursdays, supplementing with a one-hour yoga class on Saturdays.

Stick to your yoga schedule faithfully. Remember tapas, the niyama about self-discipline? Even with the best intentions, though, life can throw you curve balls that keep you from making yoga a habit. Give yourself little rewards on the days you do yoga, such as a nice breakfast or a long bubble bath. Link your yoga practice with a relaxation ritual, such as sipping tea while you watch the sun rise.

Also know that you can do yoga in mini-sessions. Do three 10-minute slots spread through the day. Use the first for warm-ups, the second for more strenuous poses, and the third for relaxation. (Of course, if your mini-sessions are a few hours apart, you'll need to warm up again going into more strenuous poses.) Do Mountain pose in the shower, or do Tree pose while you are waiting for the pasta to boil. Break up your coffee break or your lunch hour with a yoga pose minute (or two or three!).

The most spiritual time of day and the most ideal for practicing yoga is just before sunrise (about 5:30 A.M.). If you make it a habit to practice yoga before sunrise and then relax with a cup of herbal tea to watch the dawn, you'll find a new sense of peace pervading your days. And to think you've been sleeping through all that beauty!

Essential Yoga Basics

When setting up a practice at home, don't forget that every yoga practice should include the following:

- **A warm-up.** It's important to get your muscles warm and activated before you start stretching them. Warm-ups help prevent injury and make a wonderful transition from daily life to yoga mode.

- **A balanced set of poses.** Poses that bend or twist to one side should be balanced with poses that bend or twist to the other side. Forward bends balance backbends. Right-side-up poses balance inverted poses. Poses that stretch and expand are balanced by poses that curl and contract. Energizing poses balance relaxing poses. You get the idea.

- **Pranayama, or breathing exercises.** Use breath to move into a pose—and to bring that prana to you.

- **Dhyana, or meditation.** It's a good idea to blend meditation in your workout.

- **Relaxation.** *Shavasana*, or Corpse pose, should close every yoga session. This relaxation pose is so essential that we devoted a whole chapter to it, Chapter 12.

Know Your Sanskrit

Shavasana (*shava* means corpse) is perhaps the most important of all yoga asanas. This pose involves total relaxation while lying, corpse-like, on the floor. Shavasana, sometimes spelled as savasana, is a surprisingly challenging pose. It requires a full body scan to relax deeper and deeper, bringing your body, and your mind, into stillness.

When practicing poses at home on your own, keep in mind these five steps to every pose:

1. Visualize your body holding the pose.
2. Gracefully flow into the pose.
3. Become one with the pose. Find the peace and balance.
4. Gracefully flow out of the pose.
5. Reflect and release. Let go. Feel the silence.

These simple principles can be applied to any style of yoga workout. In the next chapter, we'll show you how to optimize each workout so you're getting the most out of yoga.

The Least You Need to Know

- Yoga is best learned from a good teacher. Finding a teacher who is right for your personality is important for a successful yoga practice.

- You can also learn yoga at home through books, videos, CDs or audiotapes, and the Internet.

- Establish a plan that works for you—how often you will practice yoga and what you will do in each practice.

- You can easily fit in short yoga practices throughout your day.

In This Chapter

- ◆ Guidelines for yoga practice
- ◆ Yoga's subtle challenges
- ◆ Breath-savvy yoga practices
- ◆ Benefits for your fitness regimen

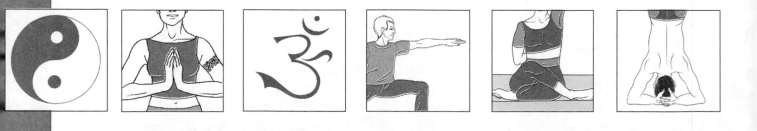

Chapter **5**

Optimize Your Yoga Workout

Before we go into the poses, we want to give you some building blocks that are assured to give you the most effective yoga workout. We'll deepen your understanding of the role breath plays in enhancing each pose, and we'll also show you how yoga can work hand in hand with the other exercises in your fitness regimen.

As you move deeper into your yoga practice, you'll discover that there are certain ground rules of practicing the asanas that hold true universally. The more your bodymind moves in tune with these yoga truths, the more profound and meaningful they will become as a complement to strengthen your yoga practice. You will find that you begin to breathe and move in all that you do with an awareness of centered balance, concentration, and subtle focus.

Yoga Ground Rules

First, let's look at some general rules for poses. Use these guidelines, and you'll find building a yoga workout is easy to do. We will remind you throughout this book to listen to your body. Pay attention to how your body is responding to each pose. Focus on how you feel in the pose. Listening to your body and responding to its needs is the best way to get the most out of each yoga pose.

Breathe and Hold Poses Peacefully

Breathe and hold poses with comfort and confidence:

◆ Hold each pose for three breath cycles (one cycle = one inhalation and one exhalation). That's to start. You may want to gradually increase the time you hold the pose and the number of breath cycles.

◆ Don't feel you have to look just like the picture! More importantly, find peace within each pose, and progress as your body allows you to.

Don't rush through the poses; hold every pose for at least three controlled breaths. Can't manage a pose that looks quite like this full Triangle pose? No problem!

If your Modified Triangle pose looks more like this, with your hand resting on your knee, you are still doing the asana correctly. Stay at the edge of your body's comfort zone, without pain or distraction. Aim for peaceful concentration.

Do Counterposes to Stay Balanced

Attain balance (Remember the yoga union of yin and yang energy?) by doing counterposes and breathing in harmony:

◆ For each pose, make sure you have a counterpose to keep your body balanced.

For example, forward bends balance backbends. Child's pose (see Chapter 11) balances Fish pose (see Chapter 7), or, as in the illustration, Downward Facing Dog pose balances Upward Facing Dog pose.

◆ Generally, exhale as you go into forward bends and inhale as you go into backbends.

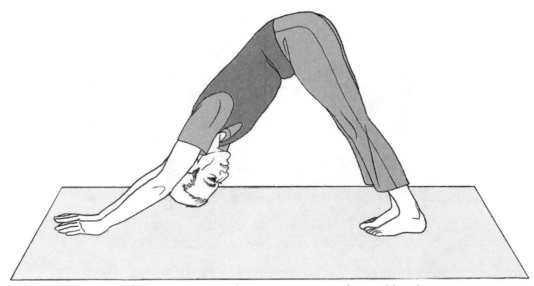

Exhale into Downward Facing Dog pose, a forward bend.

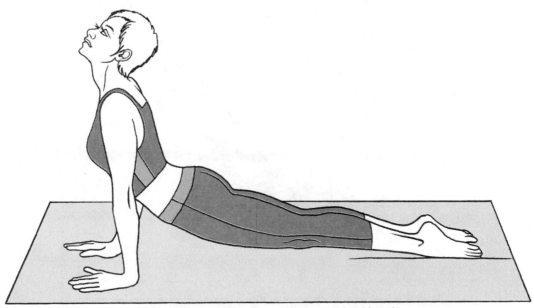

Inhale into Upward Facing Dog pose, a backbend.

Expand and Contract

Hatha Yoga is a play of contracting and expanding poses:

◆ Poses that open the body, called expansion poses, are beneficially balanced with poses that tighten the body, often called contraction poses.

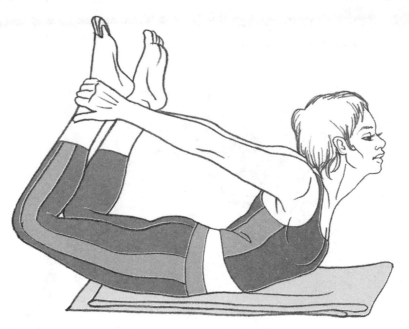

An expansion pose such as Bow pose nicely balances a contraction pose.

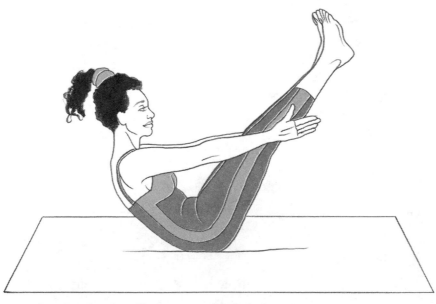

A contraction pose like Boat pose nicely balances an expansion pose.

Twistin' and Turnin'

Hatha Yoga is also a play of balancing twisting and turning poses:

◆ A twist to the left is balanced by repeating the pose with a twist to the right. Always try to do both sides—avoid favoring favorites and give both sides equal time!

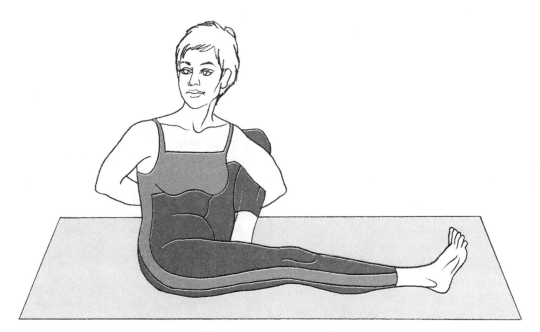

When you twist one way ...

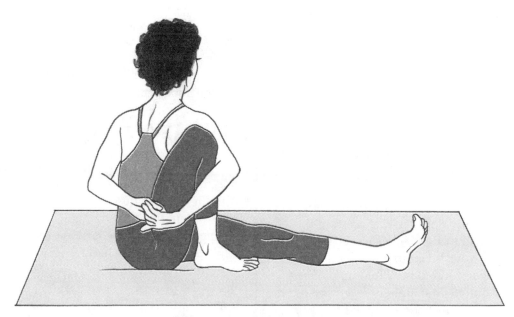

... remember to twist the other way, too.

Finding the Edge vs. Feeling the Burn

We know we have assured you yoga is easy on your body, but believe us, it is a workout. It can even be downright difficult. Just because the sensibility of yoga is nonviolence (meaning it's not harsh to your body) doesn't mean it's not challenging. Yoga can be intense.

Ouch! _____

If you happen to overdo it during your yoga workout and find yourself in serious pain, do yourself a favor and *go to your health-care provider immediately!* Ignoring the pain won't make it go away and, in some cases, could result in a serious or chronic health problem. Just do it!

The difference between yoga and other types of exercise is that the challenge and the progression are deeply internal and subtle. Here's an example: let's say you're doing a standing forward bend, trying to touch your head to your knees. The first time you try it, you don't even come close. You can barely bend forward without your back causing you pain. So bend your knees and slowly work at bending at the hip joint. Place your hands at the point where the femur (large upper leg bone) joins into the hip bone. Focus on bending forward from here instead of the waist. Slowly build so that your back strengthens and you can feel your spine lengthen as you move forward. Push in at the hips, and lean into your farthest point in the stretch and hold it. Remember to keep breathing, directing your breath through your body to the tight places in the pose. Holding the pose won't hurt, but you'll definitely feel something. Your muscles might shake a bit, and that's okay, as long as you aren't forcing the issue. Your muscles are waking up and saying, "Hey! What

is it you want us to do? This is weird, but okay, we'll give it a try." Your mind is waking up, too, and taking notice. The next time you try this pose, you may find the farthest point of the stretch is now a little farther than it was before. You stretch to this point and hold it. Now your muscles have become accustomed to a new "normal" level of flexibility. You play with the new edge and test it—not to the point of pain, but just to see where it now lies. Your muscles feel it, and so does your mind.

Build on this over a few weeks or months, and ... wow! There it is! Suddenly your head is resting quite easily on your knees. You've stretched your boundaries and pushed your edge to a new level. At this point, you may simply feel triumphant, but you may also feel an awakening to a new level of yourself. No longer simply proud of your achievement, you're now aware of yourself in a new way.

Therein lies yoga's power—the physical process breaking into the mental process and lifting the whole of you to higher and higher states of awareness.

Keep in mind that every posture contains an "edge" or a point past which—for today, at least—you can't quite go. This is the point around which you want to linger, because it's the source of yoga's power. You'll soon see how productive it is to recognize an edge but not let it define you.

More About Prana: Breathe

And once again, we remind you of your ever-present breath, prana, the universal life force. Although breathing exercises are performed separately from the poses, breathing is also important during the poses. Of course, you have to breathe while exercising, but becoming aware of your breath, even breathing in a specific way according to the posture you are holding, will enhance your practice and help your body work better. Here are a few more advanced breath-savvy concepts to keep in mind while practicing your asanas.

Ouch!

If you become out of breath or fatigued during your workout, stop! Yoga isn't circuit-training, marathon-running, or nonstop anything. Rest is encouraged within a workout—as a transition from one pose to another, as a chance to feel the aftereffects of a pose, and to maintain awareness.

Moving In and Out

Prana moves into the body when a pose opens and out of the body when a pose tightens or closes inward.

◆ Inhalation most often occurs when your chest opens, your limbs extend outward or upward, and your head is up.

◆ Exhalation most often occurs when your chest contracts inward, your limbs move close to your body, your head is down, and your body curls into itself.

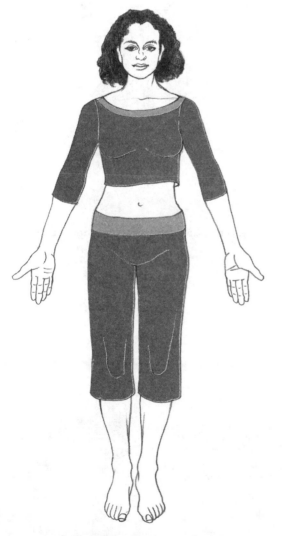

Inhale while opening your body.

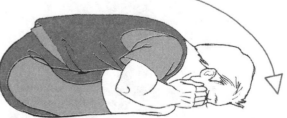

Exhale while folding the body into Butterfly pose.

Energizing and Holding Energy

When doing yoga poses, the act of holding the breath can energize prana in the body, while building endurance and strength through stillness and concentration of the bodymind on the pose.

◆ Retaining the breath after an inhalation helps stabilize and energize the chest area.

◆ Retaining the breath after an exhalation helps stabilize and energize the abdominal area and releases toxins from the body.

◆ Forward-bending poses are conducive to exhalation, then retention.

◆ Back-bending poses are conducive to inhalation, then retention.

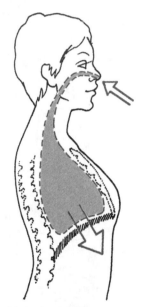
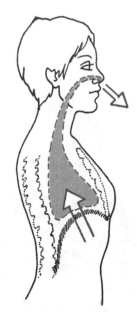

Inhale and hold the breath for a moment to energize the chest. Exhale and hold before inhaling again to energize the abdomen.

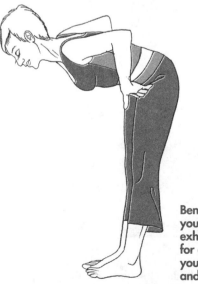

Bend forward from your hips as you exhale, then hold for a moment to feel your body's stillness and strength.

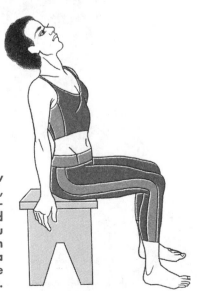

Place a stool a few inches from a wall, or use a hard-backed chair and bend back as you inhale, then retain the breath for a moment to feel the power of prana.

Breathing deeply and well during exercise keeps a steady supply of oxygen in the blood so muscles can work at their peak. Breathing keeps the mind calm and focused, which will further enhance your workout. And because the breath is the vehicle by which prana, the universal life force, enters the body, you'll certainly want to breathe deeply during your workout. Prana is the energy that keeps you vibrant and animated. It's the key to a great workout, so get as much into you as possible! Breathe! Breathe! Breathe!

Wise Yogi Tells Us

Your breath has four modes:

- Inhalation
- Retained breath after inhalation
- Exhalation
- Retained breath after exhalation

Learning how to use each mode when it is most beneficial will greatly enhance your practice.

Yoga and the Rest of Your Fitness Regimen

If you are already athletic, you'll find that yoga can improve your performance dramatically, from strength to flexibility to balance. Here's a look at how:

- **Awesome aerobics.** Yoga is a terrific complement to aerobics because it balances the frenetic energy of aerobics with a sense of calm and inner control. It can also improve your balance. The sequence of moving from Downward Dog to Upward Dog and back again can improve your aerobic performance by strengthening your body, particularly your back, legs, and upper arms. It helps build grace as the movement of the legs shift the balance of the foot from the top of the foot to the toes. It balances strength of upper body with lower body.

- **Rockin' running.** Yoga gives you flexibility, which protects from injury. It also builds strength in the feet, ankles, knees, and hips—areas where runners are injury-prone. Yoga also improves your breathing; runners tend to have shallow, hard breathing patterns. Yoga's deep-breathing exercises increase your lung capacity, getting more oxygen to your brain and increasing your endurance. Yoga is kinder to your body than running, so it makes a great alternate workout to give your body a rest from the constant pounding and joint stress runners experience.

  All variations on the Warrior poses are good for runners, because they strengthen the knees and quadriceps.

- **Biking and beyond.** Cycling is an excellent way to strengthen leg muscles without stress on joints, increase cardiovascular functioning, and spend time in the great outdoors. But while cycling is great for your leg muscles, it does very little to increase upper body strength. That's where yoga can balance out cycling by strengthening your arms and shoulders while also lengthening and loosening tight quadriceps and hamstrings (the muscles on the front and back of your thighs).

  For increased cycling performance, try Revolved Triangle pose. Revolved Triangle helps open the chest area and provides an excellent spinal twist. It also stretches your hamstrings.

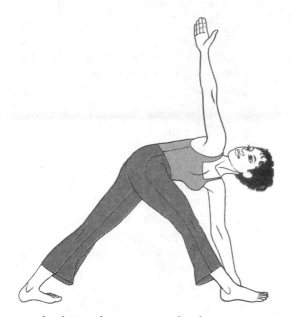

Revolved Triangle pose opens the chest, activates the spine, and stretches the hamstrings for stronger, more flexible, and more comfortable cycling.

◆ **Super-charged stretching.** The main difference between yoga and stretching is that yoga stretches are specifically designed not only to lengthen your muscles, but also to stabilize your joints, stimulate your organs, balance your endocrine system, and strengthen your muscles as you hold the stretch. It's still a good idea to do basic stretches before and especially after engaging in strenuous exercise, such as running or swimming, but if you also add yoga to your fitness program, stretching will soon be a breeze.

For increased flexibility, particularly as a warm-up and cool-down before strenuous exercise, try Lying Down Spinal Twist. This pose helps create a more supple spine, ready to stretch and move in various directions. It also limbers the neck and opens the chest. After you do this pose lying down, try doing it sitting up.

◆ **Superior swimming.** Swimming is an excellent exercise because it works your muscles and your heart without putting stress on your body. Swimming is essentially a cardiovascular exercise as well as a strength-builder. If you're a swimmer, you'll find yoga a great addition to your fitness program, because the increased flexibility and strength gained through yoga make swimming easier. Also, the breathing practices of yoga are of exceptional benefit to swimmers, who must have good control over their breath in the water.

For improved swimming performance, try Boat pose in the pool holding on to a pool ladder. Modify the angle according to your comfort level. This pose helps stretch your legs, arms, and spine for easier swimming.

◆ **Uplifting weightlifting.** Lifting weights adds strength to both muscles and bone. More and more studies suggest that weightlifting is extremely beneficial, particularly for women and seniors, to fight bone loss and muscle atrophy, keep the body in good shape, and boost metabolism. That's a plus because the more muscle mass you have, the more fat you burn even when you are just sitting at your computer. The downside of weightlifting, however, is that weightlifting alone decreases flexibility. Enter yoga.

Yoga is really a form of weightlifting, because you lift your own body weight, and that can be quite a bit of weight, particularly during the holidays. Still, if you enjoy lifting weights in addition to your own, a stretching-oriented yoga workout provides the perfect combination of strength and stretch. Try the Cow pose to complement a triceps weightlifting workout.

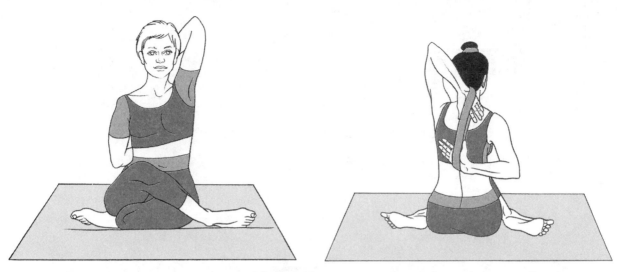

Cow pose is the perfect yoga complement to a weightlifting triceps workout. After each set, spend a minute or two in Cow pose to stretch your strengthened triceps.

A Yoga Minute

According to the National Sporting Good Association, exercise walking was the number-one fitness activity in 2004, with 84.7 million participants over age 7. The sport that grew in popularity the most? Archery!

Yoga Union

The Western approach to yoga tends to be more fitness-oriented, while the Eastern approach to yoga is based on the idea that a healthy body makes it easier to progress spiritually. Either approach benefits both body and mind. Whether you're interested in yoga for its physical benefits or for spiritual growth, you can consider the "centeredness" you achieve a splendid bonus.

The Least You Need to Know

- Though yoga is easy on your body, it is challenging. The challenge is intense, subtle, and internal.
- Use counterposes to balance each pose.
- Breathe deeply during yoga poses to keep a steady supply of oxygen in the blood allowing muscles to work at their peak.
- Yoga makes you a better runner, cyclist, dancer, swimmer, weightlifter, and all-around great athlete.

In This Part

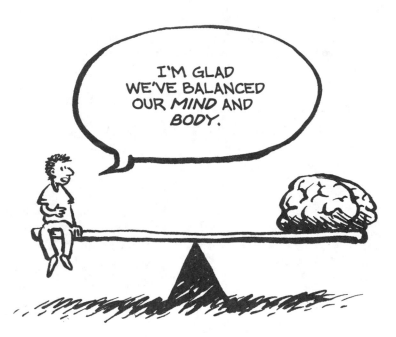

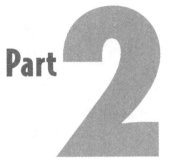

Part 2

Strength: Postures to Build Endurance

On to the workout! Part 2 consists of energizing poses you can try, master, and incorporate into your workout. Standing poses build strength, endurance, and steadiness. Balance poses improve poise and self-possession. Backbends release the flow of energy through your body. Twists and inversions rejuvenate and revitalize you. We'll give you lots of pictures and detailed descriptions so you know exactly how to do these strengthening and energizing yoga postures safely, accurately, and in the best design for bodymind balance. Let's go!

In This Chapter

◆ The importance of standing poses

◆ Mountain pose, the foundation of standing poses

◆ Triangle pose: come on, get happy!

◆ Lots more standing poses to try: Side Angle Stretch, Warrior, Lightning Bolt, and more!

◆ Balance poses, too: Tree, Eagle, Plank, Arm Balance, and more!

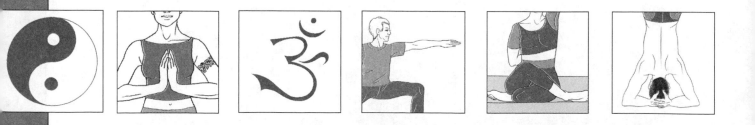

Chapter 6

What Do You Stand For?

Standing poses are essential to yoga, and Mountain pose begins the foundation. As you practice the standing poses, you'll find them becoming a good percentage of your practice. Balance, too, is integral to yoga, and is even embedded in the name of Hatha Yoga, as in *ha* and *tha*, the two sides of your body.

But standing balance poses do more than coordinate your left and right sides. They help tie your entire body and mind together into a more integrated and fully functioning body-mind whole. Balance poses also increase self-confidence, because they teach you to stay centered, calm, and strong in precarious circumstances. When you accomplish poses such as Warrior 3, you'll feel great. And that's just a taste of the power that's yet to come.

So let's get right to it!

Tadasana: Mountain Pose

Mountain pose is deceptively simple, but it's not just standing. It requires great concentration because it's easy to drift in awareness as you balance your entire body. *Tada* means "mountain," and *sana* means "straight," so tadasana (*tah-DAH-sah-nah*) means standing straight like a mountain. As you stand in tadasana, try to feel the firmness and stability of a mountain.

The balance and good posture you practice with Mountain pose lead to internal balance. Distribute your weight evenly between your heels and toes, between each leg, and over each hip. Think *balance*. Let your belly expand while the tailbone tucks under, maintaining the support of your spine. Release tensions with each inhalation.

1. Put your feet together with your toes pointed forward. Your arms should hang by your sides with your palms facing toward your body.

2. Lift your toes off the ground. Notice how the arches of your feet feel. Lift up slightly. Now, slowly place each toe back on the ground while you maintain the feeling of the lift in your arches. Feel the lift all the way up your entire body.

3. Feel your spine and the back of your neck lengthening. (Remember that string pulling up the crown of your head?) Pull up your thigh muscles and lift the front of your body. Relax your hands and face.

Ouch!

When holding Mountain pose, tilt your tailbone under, allowing your pelvis to slightly tilt inward. This movement will naturally tilt your stomach back toward your spine. The heels on our shoes (even on our gym shoes!) constantly push our hips back and our stomachs out. Realign them with tadasana.

Continuing the Challenge: Visualization

Visualization is an effective tool for many poses, but especially Mountain pose. As you hold this pose, imagine you are a mountain. Feel how steady, strong, solid, and balanced you are.

Continuing the Challenge: Namaste, or Prayer Pose

To give your shoulders, elbows, wrists, and upper arm muscles a nice stretch, try Mountain pose with your hands in prayer position, also called namaste, behind your back. Start by bringing your hands behind you at about hip level and touching your fingertips together. Gradually move your palms together so your fingers point up behind your back, and slide your hands up as far as is comfortable. The more you do this pose, the higher up you'll be able to bring your hands and the more flexibility you'll enjoy in your shoulder joints.

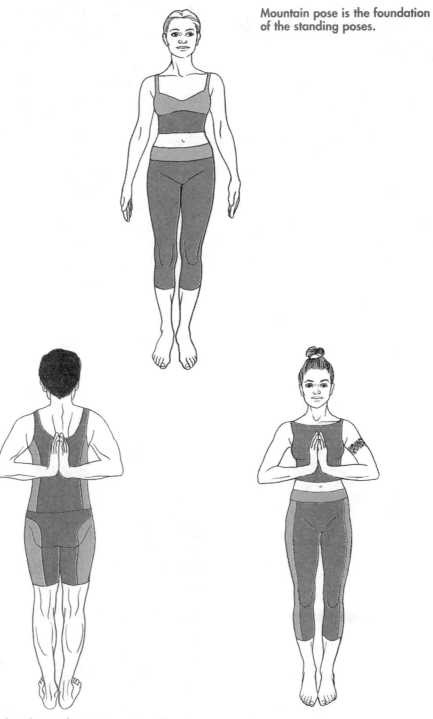

Mountain pose is the foundation of the standing poses.

Holding your hands together in Prayer pose, or namaste, behind your back while in Mountain pose adds balance, reverence, and a nice shoulder stretch to this basic pose.

Prayer pose brings peace.

Trikonasana: Triangle, the Happy Pose

Forming triangles with your body will teach it a sense of direction. The basic triangle, or trikonasana (*trih-koh-NAH-sah-nah*), is known as the happy pose because it opens your Venus chakra (the energy center located behind your heart) and allows joy to fill your body and radiate within you and from you. Trikonasana tones your spine and waist. It stimulates your bowels and intestines, strengthens your legs and ankles, improves your circulation, and develops your chest. It also strengthens your breath.

1. Stand with your feet about three feet apart, your right foot pointed forward, your left foot turned out comfortably, about 90 degrees.

2. Bend to the left, reaching your left arm toward your left foot, and stretching your right arm straight up over your head. If you can, rest your left hand on your left ankle or calf.

3. Look straight ahead or toward the sky and stretch your neck. Feel the triangle formed by your legs and the ground, as well as the triangle shape formed by your entire body. Breathe deeply.

4. Slowly come back to a standing position, then repeat on the other side.

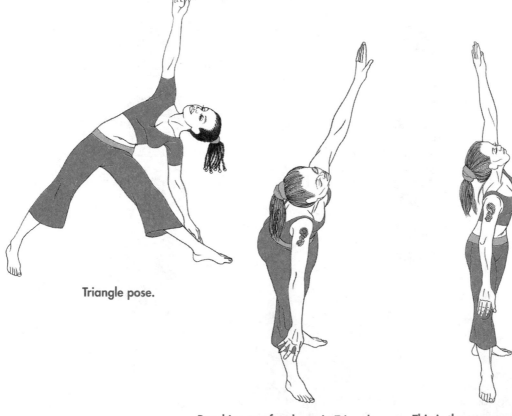

Triangle pose.

Reaching too far down in Triangle can throw your body out of alignment by pulling your hips back.

This is the proper alignment of Triangle pose. Notice how the hip and pelvis are pulled in and aligned with the rest of the body.

Easing into the Pose: Standing Side Bend

For those of you new to yoga, first try Standing Side Bend to prepare your body for Triangle. This pose has all the benefits of Triangle but is less intense. Once your torso feels more flexible and strong, move gradually into Triangle pose, moving down only as far as your body will comfortably allow.

Modified Triangle

As you ease into Triangle, don't worry if you can't reach your ankle at first. The length of your stretch doesn't equal the quality of your yoga. Don't be so eager to touch your ankle that you tilt your body forward, cutting off your body's energy flow. Pretend your shoulders remain pressed against an invisible wall behind you. You'll stay aligned and your energy will soar!

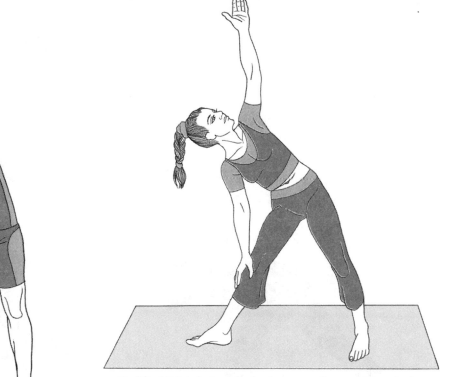

Modified Triangle is a perfectly correct form of Triangle for beginners. The more flexible your torso and shoulders become, the farther down toward the floor you can move.

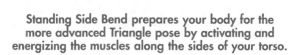

Standing Side Bend prepares your body for the more advanced Triangle pose by activating and energizing the muscles along the sides of your torso.

Continuing the Challenge: Revolved Triangle Pose

Take the Triangle pose a step further with the Revolved Triangle pose. After holding Triangle for a few breaths, switch arms. Bring the raised arm down, and hold the other side of your calf or ankle. Bring the other arm straight up above you. Breathe, then return to Mountain pose, and repeat on the other side.

A Yoga Minute

The triangle is used as a spiritual symbol in many different cultures, from the goddess tradition (virgin, mother, and crone) to Christianity (Father, Son, and Holy Ghost). In ancient Egypt, it represented the female principle, motherhood, and the moon. In Arabia, the triangle symbolized the three lunar Goddesses, while the Celtic shamrock was a three-way design originally representing the three mothers. The double triangle symbolizes creation in the Tantric tradition, with the downward-pointing triangle representing the feminine and the upward-pointing triangle symbolizing the masculine. But consider also the triangular relationship of body, mind, and spirit.

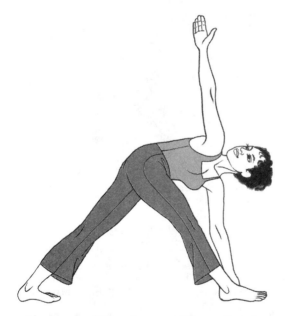

The Revolved Triangle pose might, at first glance, look like the regular Triangle pose, but look closer. The body is twisted around so the left hand is by the right foot. This is considered a more difficult pose because it incorporates a full spinal twist into the Triangle.

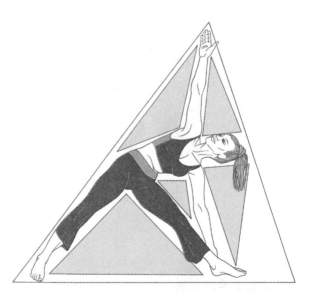

How many triangles can you find in this picture? Look at the lines made by the body and those suggested by the body. Perhaps you can find more than we did.

Parshvakonasana: Side Angle Stretch

Parshva means "flank" or "side," and *kona* means "angle"—hence, parshvakonasana (*par-shvah-KOH-nah-sah-nah*) means Side Angle Stretch! This pose tones your legs, strengthens your knees, and lengthens your spine. It relieves back pain and sciatica problems, and stretches and strengthens the hips and stomach.

Exhale as you go into this pose, and inhale as you come out; breathe while you hold the pose.

1. Stand with your feet three to four feet apart. Point your left foot forward and turn your right foot out so it is perpendicular to the left, the right heel lined up with the arch of the left foot.

2. Bend your right knee into a right angle with the floor and lean into the stretch so that the right side of your body moves toward the top of your right thigh and your right hand reaches toward the ground beside your right foot. Don't worry about touching the floor with your hand. Instead, concentrate on the side stretch of your body.

3. Stretch your left arm over your head so it forms a relatively straight line with your left leg and torso. Your left palm should face downward. Look up toward your arm and feel the stretch from your toes into your fingertips. Breathe deeply.

4. Return to Mountain pose, then repeat on the other side.

Ouch! _____

In Side Angle Stretch, be careful not to overextend your bent knee. It should be at or nearly at a right angle to the floor. Also, don't let your back leg flop. Keep it active by pushing down on your back heel.

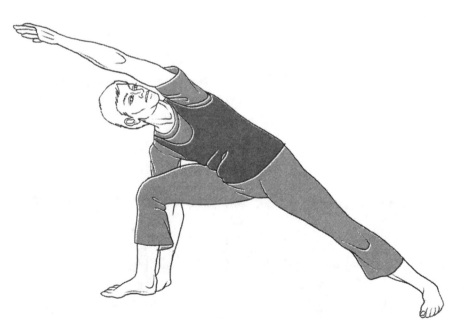

Side Angle Stretch pose.

Virabhadrasana: Warrior 1 Pose

It takes the tremendous strength of a warrior to "conquer" inner peace. The Warrior pose, or virabhadrasana (*vee-rab-hah-DRAH-sah-nah*), fills the body with nobility and strength, calling upon the power and nourishment of the sun while firmly planting the feet upon the earth. *Vira* means "hero," and *bhadra* means "auspicious," so virabhadrasana means "heroic auspicious posture."

There are three variations of Warrior, and we'll start with Warrior 1. This pose aids in deep breathing, relieves a stiff neck and shoulders, strengthens the legs, and trims the hips.

Be sure to exhale as you go into Warrior 1, and inhale as you go out of the pose. Be careful to relax your muscles while in Warrior 1. Keep your face and neck relaxed. Breathe normally. Feel the warrior strength gathering inside you.

1. From Mountain pose, step your right foot three to four feet back. Angle your right foot out so that your right arch is in line with your left heel.

2. Raise both arms over your head with your palms facing each other. Look straight ahead or upward at your hands. If your shoulders are relaxed, bring your palms together. For those with tight shoulders, it's best to keep your hands apart, which will help your shoulders stay down away from your ears.

3. Bend your left knee so that your thigh and calf form a right angle. Rotate your body to the left, directly in line with your left leg. Keep your back foot firmly planted and your back leg straight. Push down on your back heel. Take three rich, full breaths.

4. Return to the starting position and repeat on the other side.

Easing into the Pose: Arching

Remember that lift of your arches in Mountain pose? Notice what happens when you apply that technique here. Lift the toes of your back foot. Watch your arch slightly lift. Slowly place your toes back on the ground while maintaining the lift in the arch. As your toes touch the ground, let the lift of your arch ascend throughout the rest of your body. Breathe.

Continuing the Challenge: Intensifying Your Strength

Bring your palms together and interlace your fingers over your head, while keeping your index fingers pointed straight up. Keep your shoulders down, away from your ears. Look up at your hands while keeping your neck strong. Imagine strength and energy shooting out of the tips of your fingers. This variation intensifies the strength and energy of the Warrior 1.

Warrior 2

Warrior 2 builds on the benefits of Warrior 1, strengthening and shaping your legs. It also can relieve leg cramps, bring flexibility to the legs and back, tone your abdomen, and strengthen your ankles and arms.

1. Begin as for Warrior 1. Keep your upper body facing forward as you bend your left leg into or close to a right angle with the floor.

2. Lift both arms straight out to form a "T" shape with your body. Look toward your left arm. Keep your shoulders down.

3. Hold the pose for at least a few breaths, return to the starting position, then repeat on the other side.

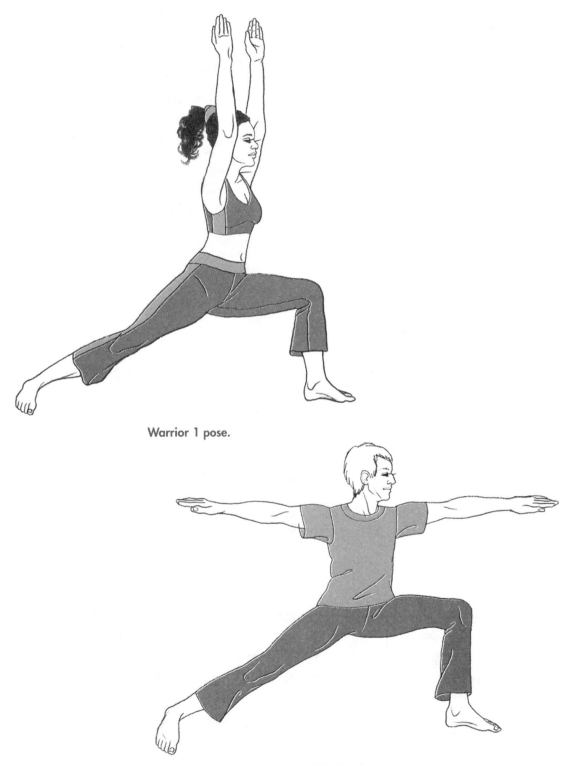

Warrior 1 pose.

Warrior 2 pose.

Warrior 3

Warrior 3 develops the strength and shape of your legs and abdomen; it also gives you agility, poise, better concentration, and improved balance. It is a more difficult pose than the first two Warrior poses.

Work on extending the amount of time you can hold this pose, for a superpowered, strength-building, balance-honing workout. Watch your breath! As the breath comes into balance, so do the balance poses. Don't hold your breath. Keep breathing, slowly and steadily.

1. Assume Warrior 1, then lean forward slightly, slowly straightening your front leg as you lift your back leg.

2. Extend your arms in front of you with your palms together, looking toward your hands. Work toward bringing your arms and lifted leg perpendicular to the floor. If you can't do that at first, no problem. This is something you will be able to do when you have gained sufficient strength and balance.

3. Return to a neutral position, then repeat on the opposite side.

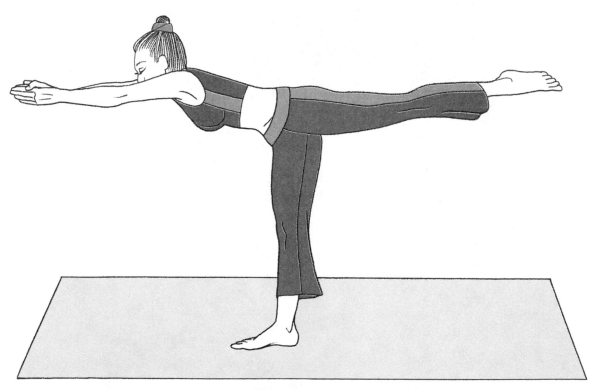

Warrior 3 pose.

Continuing the Challenge: A Warrior Vinyasana

Combine Mountain, Warrior 1, Warrior 2, and Triangle into a vinyasana, or a flowing sequence. It's a great way to get your heart pumping and to energize your body and mind for a challenging day. Begin in Mountain, then flow into Warrior 1. From Warrior 1, rotate your torso and bring your arms down into Warrior 2 position, then flow into Triangle pose, and back into Mountain.

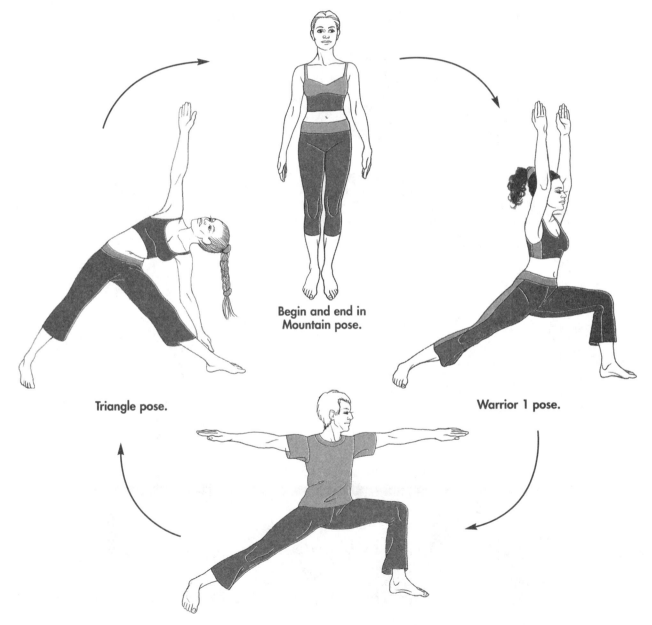

Begin and end in Mountain pose.

Triangle pose.

Warrior 1 pose.

Warrior 2 pose.

Continuing the Challenge: Three Warriors

Once you've combined these, add Warrior 3 to the sequence, flowing from Warrior 1 to Warrior 3, Warrior 2 to Triangle, back to Mountain pose; then turn the other direction, and start all over again on the other side. Combining the warriors as 1-3-2 makes for an especially graceful transition between poses. This Warrior sequence is a real confidence builder. For more vinyasanas see Part 5.

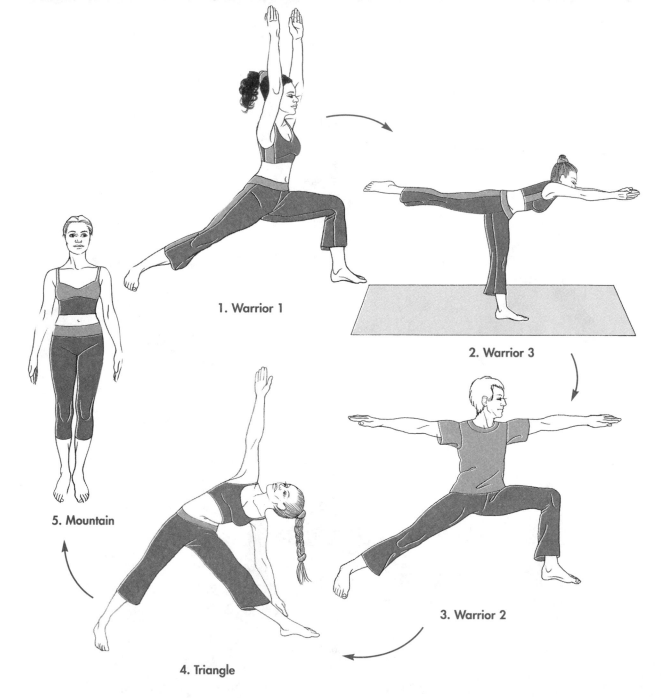

1. Warrior 1

2. Warrior 3

5. Mountain

3. Warrior 2

4. Triangle

Natarajasana: Shiva Pose

This beautiful but challenging balance pose is named after the Hindu god Shiva, whose every step destroys and then subsequently recreates the universe. Shiva is sometimes called the cosmic dancer, and this pose is sometimes called Dancer pose.

1. Begin in Mountain pose. Bend one knee and grasp this leg's ankle behind you. Raise your opposite arm above you for balance.

2. Slowly bend forward and pull gently on your ankle so your raised leg extends behind you, knee bent so your foot points upward.

3. Counter the balance by lowering your extended arm in front of you so that as your leg moves back, your arm moves in front.

Easing into the Pose: Visualization

As you begin in Mountain pose, visualize a steady and firmly rooted center. As you hold this pose, visualize the ebb and flow of the universe. Visualize holding yourself calmly in the continual flux of the universe, through the cycles of creation and destruction.

Continuing the Challenge

Once you are very secure in this pose, you can reach both hands behind you to grasp your foot.

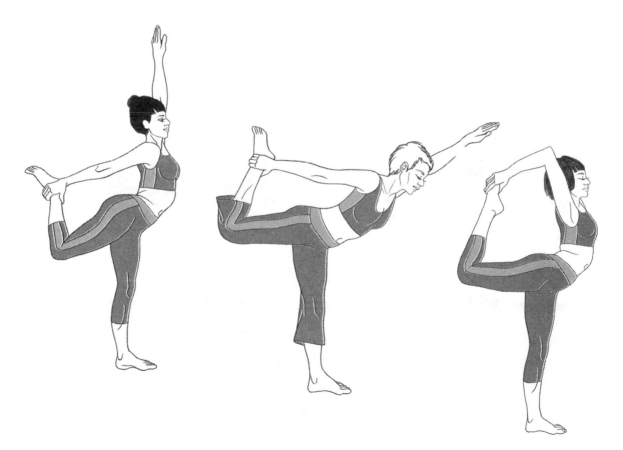

Shiva pose, sometimes called Dancer pose, can be done at any of three levels of intensity.

Utkatasana: Lightning Bolt Pose

Lightning Bolt pose, or utkatasana (*oot-kah-TAH-sah-nah*), is a powerful pose. Utkatasana means "raised posture." As you form the shape of a lightning bolt, you are filled with the dynamic energy of lightning. Utkatasana removes shoulder stiffness, strengthens your legs and ankles, lifts your diaphragm, massages your heart, tones your back and stomach, and develops your chest. It also warms up your body.

1. Begin in tadasana, Mountain pose.
2. Separate your feet hip distance apart.
3. In one flowing movement, bend your knees as you lift your arms over your head with palms facing in. Bend forward at the hips keeping the spine straight. Fully engage your thigh muscles to keep your knees from buckling inward.
4. Extend your arms so they are straight and in line with your ears. Feel the shape of the lightning bolt and breathe deeply.
5. Return to tadasana.

Lightning Bolt pose.

Standing Forward Stretch opens the chest and shoulders while stretching the hamstrings.

Continuing the Challenge: Squat on Heels and Toes

Vary Lightning Bolt by turning it into a "Squat on Heels and Toes" pose. Stand with your feet hip distance apart. Squat, first standing on your toes, then squatting down. Come back up into Mountain pose. Next time, try squatting down while keeping your heels on the floor. This is more difficult, because it requires a fuller stretch of your quadriceps. These squatting variations develop the ankles, knees, and arches, while deeply stretching the quadriceps and knee joints. Be careful to keep your knees over your ankles. Don't let them droop in or out as you bend.

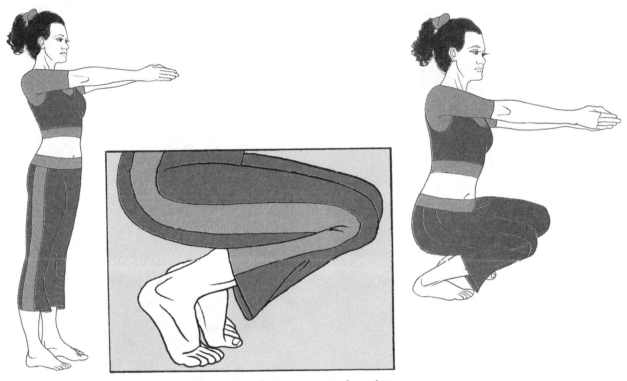

Moving into the Squat on Heels and Toes pose.

Plank Pose

Now let's try getting down on the floor for a whole new angle on balance poses. The Plank pose develops strength in your arms and legs. It helps create a balanced and strong body. It is often used as a transition pose, leading or connecting one pose to another.

1. Begin in Downward Facing Dog, as shown in Chapter 5. (This foundational pose of yoga is explained further in Chapter 11.)

2. Exhale as you lower your hips down so that your body is in a straight line from your head to your ankles.

3. Try to keep your body in a straight line from your ears to your ankles. You will discover where the weakest areas of your body are the longer you hold this position: they are the parts that start to sag toward the floor!

4. Breathe. Push your heels out to keep your lower back from caving in. Don't let your torso collapse into Plank pose. Hold the pose only as long as you can with correct form.

5. Come back down onto your stomach, or use this pose as a transition into Arm Balance pose, shown in the following section.

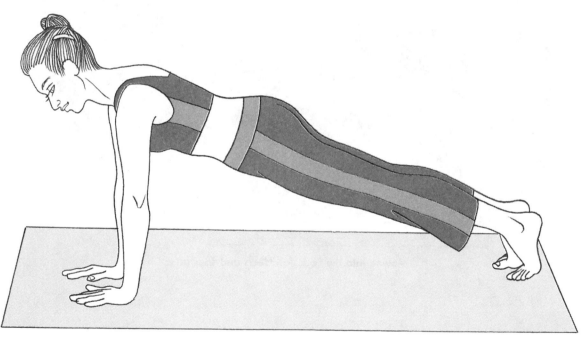

Plank pose.

Vashishthasana: Arm Balance

Vashishthasana (*VAH-shish-THAH-sah-nah*) is a pose named after the Indian sage Vashishtha. Vashishthasana strengthens the wrists and arms and tones the lumbar and coccyx regions of the spine. It also develops concentration, non-attachment to either achievement or failure, and an undisturbed, steady mind.

1. Begin in Plank pose.
2. Turn your entire body to the right, and balance on your right arm and foot on the side of your body. Your torso should be in a straight line, held in a diagonal to the floor by your right arm.
3. Lift your left arm up straight in the air with your palm facing forward.

Ouch! _____

Keep breathing steadily throughout Vashishthasana. Don't let your hips droop down, because this will cause strain to your back and put undue force on your arms. Keep your elbows straight, and keep your foot balanced on your leg. Don't let anything droop!

Easing into the Pose: Loose Limbs

Don't lock your elbow in this pose or you could injure it. Keep your arm straight, but maintain flexibility in your elbow so you could bend it easily at any time during the pose. If you find you are straining your wrist or elbow or if your arm starts to shake, stop.

Continuing the Challenge: A Variation

Try this challenging variation: from Arm Balance, slowly raise your straightened upper leg until it is parallel to the floor. Then, raise it higher and bring your raised arm down to meet your foot. Grab your toes and lift so your legs form a right angle to each other.

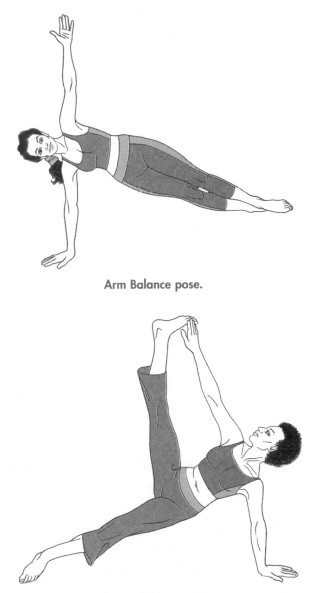

Arm Balance pose.

This variation of Arm Balance takes great strength and balance and fortifies the muscles in your arms, back, abdomen, and legs.

Vrikshasana: Tree Pose

Vrikshasana (*vrik-SHAH-sah-nah*) is one of the most basic balance poses. *Vriksha* means "tree," and a tree is soundly rooted in the earth but grows upward with branches reaching out to the sun. Wind might move the branches, but the tree stands firm. Vrikshasana tones the legs, opens the hips, and promotes physical balance. It also develops concentration and mindfulness.

Throughout vrikshasana, keep your breathing steady and regular so it doesn't interfere with your balance.

1. Begin in tadasana, Mountain pose.

2. Bring your hands together in front of your chest with your palms together in namaste (as if praying).

3. Bring your left leg up and balance the sole of your left foot on the inner thigh of your right leg, as high as you are able.

4. Raise your arms over your head, keeping your palms together. Hold a steady, forward focus with your gaze.

5. Return to tadasana, then repeat with the right leg.

Ouch!

In vrikshasana, be careful not to raise one hip higher than the other. Keep your hips even by lowering the position of your foot on your inner thigh. Bend your straight knee slightly, then straighten it to fully engage your front thigh muscle.

Easing into the Pose

If you find it too difficult to balance in tadasana, bring the sole of your foot to your opposite leg's inner calf instead of the thigh, or even rest it against your opposite ankle with toes remaining on the ground. Also, you can leave your palms apart when you raise your arms. This great separation between your hands can help you balance more easily. When you feel more confident in the pose, you can bring that foot farther up and those palms together.

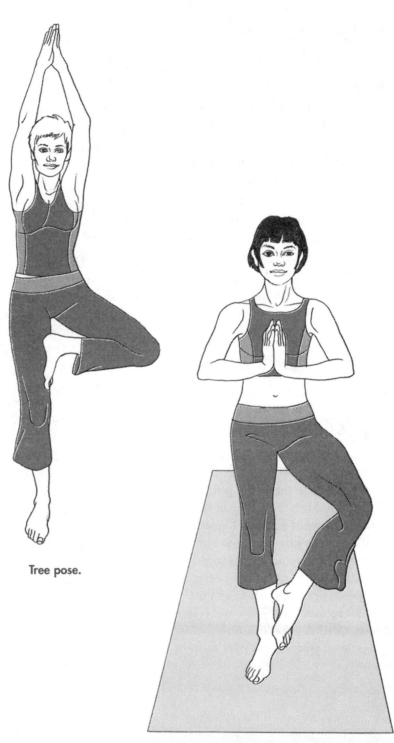

Tree pose.

If you have trouble balancing, keep your raised foot just over the ankle of your standing foot in Modified Tree pose.

Ardha Baddha Padmottanasana: Standing Half Bound Lotus Pose

This more advanced variation of the Tree pose has the same benefits as Tree pose but allows you to open your hips more fully, as well as your chest.

1. Stand with your bent right ankle resting on the front of your straight left thigh.

2. Bring your right arm behind your back and connect it to your right foot in front.

3. Lower your knee slightly toward the floor and raise your left arm over your head. Take three breaths.

4. Return to the starting position, then repeat on the other side.

Easing into the Pose: Laying the Foundation

This is a challenging pose. If your hips are not open enough yet and your knee isn't pointing toward the floor, it'll be difficult to connect your hand with your foot and could also overstrain your knee. Instead, practice the Eagle pose (following), Side Angle Stretch (earlier in this chapter), Bow pose, Upward Facing Dog, and Butterfly pose to open the hips and both Standing and Lying Down Spinal Twists to help your body prepare for the Half Bound Lotus. Practicing these poses opens the chest and increases shoulder and spinal flexibility, and you will eventually get to where you can reach your arm far enough behind you to grab your foot.

Continuing the Challenge: An Inversion

If you have mastered Standing Half Bound Lotus, add an inversion to this already challenging pose. Once secure in Standing Half Bound Lotus, exhale and slowly bend forward to place your palm on the floor next to your foot. Hold for several breaths, then slowly return to standing upright.

Continuing the Challenge: Extended Hand-to-Toe Pose

Standing Half Bound Lotus can morph into Extended Hand-to-Toe pose, another challenging balance pose. From Standing Half Bound Lotus, let go of your foot with your hand but keep your knee bent, your foot at your hip. Bring your hand around to the front and again grasp your toe. This time, slowly straighten your knee so your leg is outstretched in front of you. Lower your other hand to rest on your hip or stretch it out to the side for balance. Breathe and hold for a minute or so, then slowly release your foot and lower it back to the floor.

Once you become very secure in this pose, you can move your foot from the front to the side, but don't try this unless you are comfortable and stable with your leg in front and you're able to completely straighten your leg.

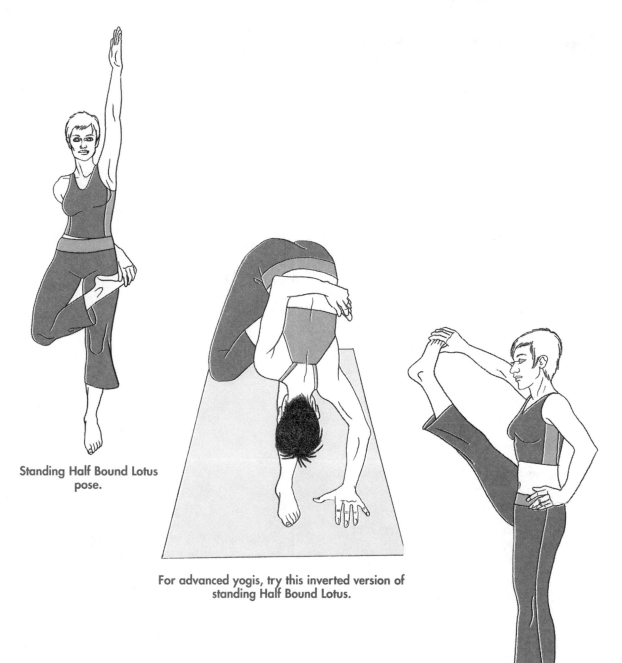

Standing Half Bound Lotus
pose.

For advanced yogis, try this inverted version of
standing Half Bound Lotus.

Extended Hand-to-Toe pose
takes strength and balance.

Garudasana: Eagle Pose

Try this pose when you are feeling mentally or physically blocked, and you just might find yourself soaring. As with the Tree pose, garudasana (*gah-roo-DAH-sah-nah*) improves balance and concentration as well as develops the ankles and removes stiffness in the shoulders.

The Eagle pose is challenging. Don't force that ankle around your standing leg, or you could injure your knee! If your ankle doesn't hook around your standing leg easily, just place the top of your foot behind your ankle or your calf of your standing leg. Eventually, your flexibility will increase.

1. Begin in tadasana, but with your knees slightly bent.

2. Bend one leg over the other like you are crossing your thighs, then hook your ankle around the back of your other ankle. Try to stay balanced between your heel and toes.

3. Bend your elbows and bring one arm under the other arm, connecting your palms in front of your face. Even though your body is twisting, imagine your torso lifting and straightening. Breathe!

4. Return to tadasana, and repeat on the other side. This pose is usually easier going one way than it is going the other way. Continue trying it both ways, and eventually you'll balance.

A Yoga Minute _____

The eagle is a sacred animal in many spiritual cultures, from Native America to ancient Hindu, and Garuda, a Hindu god, was thought to be half man and half eagle. Eagle pose is named after Garuda, who was said to be the carrier of the great Hindu god Vishnu and also the remover of obstacles.

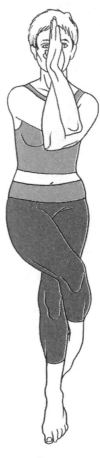

Eagle pose.

Ardha Chandrasana: Half Moon Pose

Half Moon is a beautiful pose in which your body imitates the shape of a half moon. This balance pose improves your coordination and your mental concentration, as well as helping to align your spine. You can do this pose with a yoga block or other support such as a book or small stool, or you can try it on the floor. The key is to keep your torso and limbs as straight as possible so your body and raised leg are parallel to the floor, while your arms and standing leg are perpendicular to the floor. This pose is easier to do in front of a mirror so you can check your alignment.

1. Stand in Mountain pose. Place a stool or other support (if using one) against the wall for support.

2. Inhale and open your feet so they are shoulder-width apart. Turn your left foot in and your right foot out into the foot position used for the first two Warrior poses.

3. Raise your arms straight out on either side so they are parallel to the floor.

4. Exhale and bend your right knee, placing your right palm on your thigh. Bring your left leg up as you begin to straighten your right knee. As your right knee straightens, your right hand comes down to the stool or floor.

5. Align your arms so they are perpendicular to the floor and in line with each other, as well as parallel to your standing leg. Energize the fingers of your raised hand, pointing them up.

6. Continue looking forward for balance. Keep your gaze steady on a point of focus.

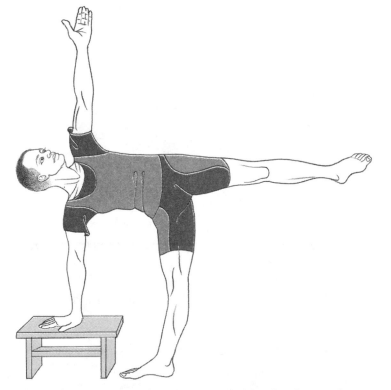

Half Moon pose takes great strength and balance and fortifies the muscles in your arms, back, abdomen, and legs.

Bhujapidasana: Crow Pose

Crow pose is the first in three series of bird poses that are extremely challenging. Crow pose looks difficult, but once you find your balance, it's really not as hard as you might think. This pose nourishes and strengthens the hands, wrists, and arms in addition to cultivating great focus.

Don't be surprised if you can't do this pose right away, or can only balance for a few seconds. The more you practice the Crow, the more confident and balanced you will become.

1. Exhale and squat down with your feet together and knees apart. Place your hands about one foot in front of your feet, fingers slightly spread, about six inches apart.

2. Gently rock back and forth on the balls of your feet to find your center of gravity.

3. Place your upper arms, right on the triceps (the muscles on the backs of your upper arms), firmly under your kneecaps. Continue to rock gently, keeping your feet on the floor, just to get a feel for where the point of your balance will be.

4. Focus on a spot on the floor just in front of your hands and gently ease your feet off the floor, resting your knees on your upper arms.

Start with Crouching pose. For this pose, squat as you would for Crow pose, with your feet together, knees apart, and hips dropped toward the floor. If possible, bring the soles of your feet all the way to the floor (this is difficult, and you might need to stay on the balls of your feet at first, which is also just fine). Reach your arms around and under your knees to grasp your ankles. Rest and breathe in this position to strengthen your legs and your ankle, knee, and hip joints.

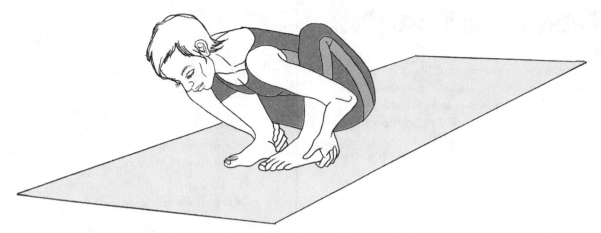

Crouching pose can help you feel more comfortable in an extreme squat before attempting a squat balancing pose like Crow pose.

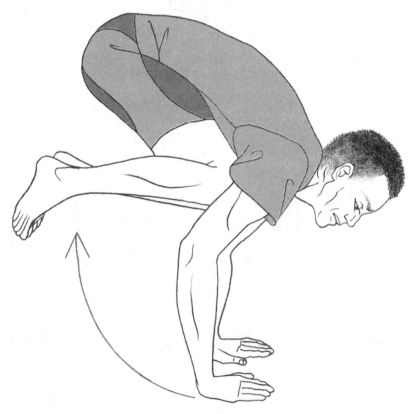

Crow pose.

Kukkutasana: Rooster Pose

In Rooster pose, your arms pierce the Lotus pose to stand on the ground like a rooster. This pose looks fancy and is lots of fun to do once you are able to master it comfortably. However, you must be able to sit comfortably in Lotus pose before attempting this pose (see Chapter 9). Rooster pose increases hip flexibility, shoulder strength, and concentration.

1. Sit in Lotus pose.

2. Slide each hand between the calf and thigh of each leg and place on the ground under your hips, rocking back to make a space. Inhale.

3. Exhale as you slowly straighten your elbows, pushing down on the floor to lift your body above the floor so your hands support your weight. You will have to adjust to find your center of balance.

4. Breathe and hold for a short time, then lower yourself back down.

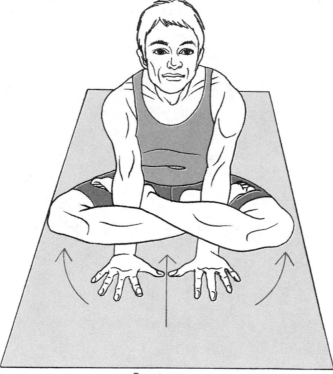

Rooster pose.

Mayurasana: Peacock Pose

Peacock pose is another challenging pose that takes great abdominal and back strength. It is great for strengthening your body's core, honing balance and concentration, and improving arm and wrist strength, but it might take quite a while to master.

This pose is particularly easy for men because men tend to have more upper body musculature. Women tend to have a lower center of gravity in the hip area, which can make this balance much more difficult to find. Women might have better luck doing the Lotus version of this pose because it brings the legs closer to the center of the body.

1. Begin by squatting down onto your knees. Place your palms on the floor together between your knees. At first, point your fingers to the side. Eventually, work toward being able to point your fingers back behind you.

2. Bend your elbows and slowly move your body forward until your elbows are over your abdomen and your upper arms hug the front of your chest. Slowly extend your legs out behind you, toes resting on the floor.

3. Easing forward, gradually and slowly move your head toward the ground until your feet lift off the ground. Keep your body, head to toe, in a straight line.

Imagine you are a teeter-totter finding that center balance. Don't try to lift your legs off the ground, just let the balance of your upper body and gravity do the work.

Journey of a Lifetime

Working toward stability and balance in your yoga practice can be a challenging and exciting journey that lasts a lifetime. Learning the basic standing postures is a great way to start, and balance poses will increase your stability. Practicing these basics will improve all aspects of your yoga practice and give you an inner peace and strength. Working toward more challenging poses keeps your yoga workout inspiring and stimulating.

The Least You Need to Know

◆ Standing poses like Mountain, Triangle, Side Angle Stretch, Warrior, and Lightning Bolt are important basics for strength and balance.

◆ Posture isn't just about looking good. It has a profound effect on your health and well-being.

◆ Practice the basic standing postures before you progress to more complicated poses.

◆ Balance poses like Tree, Eagle, Crow, Rooster, and Peacock create stability and a centered sense of being.

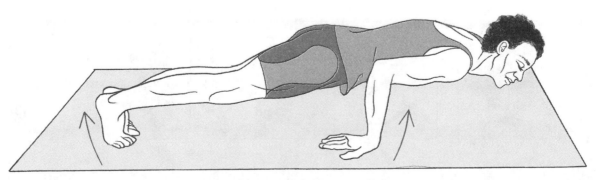

Peacock pose.

In This Chapter

◆ The health benefits of backbends

◆ Backbends help you laugh more

◆ Lots of great back-bending postures to try: Cobra, Bow, Upward Facing Dog, Fish, Camel, and Wheel

◆ Modifications, challenges, and other tips to improve your yoga practice

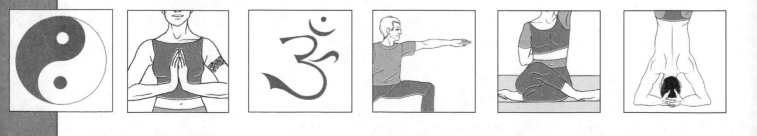

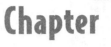

Bending Over Backbends

A few people have naturally flexible spines and find backbends easy, but for most people, backbends are a challenge. We tend to spend more of our lives bent slightly forward, and our spines just aren't used to bending the other way. All the more reason to practice backbends.

Open Up and Laugh More

Backbend poses are extremely beneficial for improving your spine and toning your internal organs. Backbend poses open your chakras, or energy centers (see Appendix B), which allows prana to flow through you and lets joy energy flow through you unimpeded. You may find that backbends are good for laughter. Really!

Before you start, perform a simple stretch to open your neck, shoulders, and chest. Sit up straight in a chair, inhale, and arch your neck back. Focus your gaze upward. Feel that openness in the center of your chest? Remember, in all backbends, avoid the impulse to crunch your neck back. *Do you feel a smile coming on?*

Bhujangasana: Cobra Pose

The Cobra pose, bhujangasana (*BOO-jhan-GAH-sah-nah*), helps align your spinal disks, open up your heart chakra, and strengthen your back. It also strengthens your nervous system and your eyes.

1. Lie on your stomach, flat on the floor, with your heels and toes together. Place your hands on the floor on both sides of your chest. Rest your forehead on the floor (you might want to use a mat for this one).

2. Inhale and lift your forehead, then your chin, then your shoulders, then your chest off the floor. Keep your hips pressed against the floor.

3. Look upward and breathe. Try sticking out your tongue and opening your mouth wide to help release your face. Then return to the starting position.

Easing into the Pose: It's the Spine, Baby

Don't rely on your arms for this pose. The secret is in lengthening your spine. To see how much you are using your arms for support, lift your palms off the floor, as you see in the drawing. How much of your body comes down? If it's a lot, your arms are doing a good portion of the work. Work on strengthening your spine before you push yourself to go higher. And remember, when practicing the Cobra pose, keep your elbows in toward the body and pull your shoulder blades down your back, being careful not to scrunch them up toward your neck.

Continuing the Challenge: Backward Boat

This variation pose looks like a canoe, but it's actually called Poorva Naukasana or the Backward Boat pose. Straighten your elbows and rest your arms alongside your body. Then, inhale and lift your arms and legs off the floor. As you hold this pose, you can slowly move your arms out to the sides, as if you are flying, and around to the front (think Superman or Superwoman!), then slowly back around to the sides and alongside the body again. This variation on Cobra is a great torso strengthener and helps balance the muscles of the lower back.

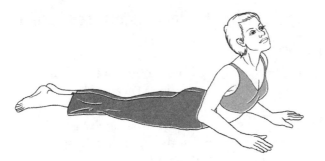

Cobra pose.

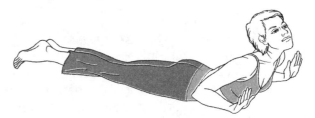

Are your arms doing more of the work than your spine? Lift your arms off the floor and make your spine work harder. Your back will thank you for it.

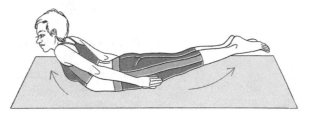

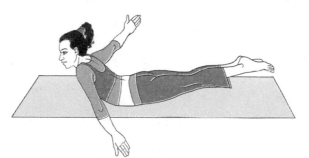

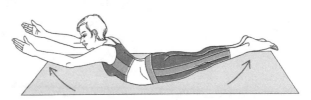

These Backward Boat variations strengthen the lower back and hone focus in preparation for Locust or Full Bow pose.

Shalabhasana: Locust Pose

Locust pose is a challenging pose that you can try after you've strengthened your back muscles with other backbend poses. Locust pose uses the core strength of the torso, particularly the back muscles, to lift the lower half of the body off the ground. This pose is an incredible lower body strengthener. It also aligns the spine and helps balance the nervous system.

If you need to work up to this one, use Single-Leg Locust pose. Keep your arms alongside your torso, palms on the floor, and just lift one leg off the floor.

1. Lie on your stomach with your chin on the floor, legs together, arms alongside your torso, and palms on the floor.

2. Slide your hands under your torso and make fists under each upper thigh with your thumb pointing down. Elbows are as close together as possible with your arms straight.

3. Inhale and energize your legs and hips, straightening them so they rise off the ground and balance on your fists.

Easing into the Pose: Single-Leg Locust Pose

This pose is a great way to get strengthening benefits before you are advanced enough to do the full Locust. Lie on your stomach as with Locust pose, but keep your arms alongside your torso, palms on the floor. Inhale, with your chin on the floor, and energize your legs and hips. Lift just one leg off the floor as high as you can without experiencing discomfort in your back. Breathe and hold for a few moments, then slowly lower the leg back to the floor. Repeat on the other side, of course!

Continuing the Challenge

Start in Locust, using your fists to balance. Continue to breathe as you lift your legs and hips off your fists and upward. Keep your chin on the floor.

 A Yoga Minute

The world is full of wise yogis—even celebrities! These celebrities have all practiced yoga: Helen Hunt, Gwyneth Paltrow, Cameron Diaz, Jerry Seinfeld, Nicholas Cage, Woody Harrelson, Charlie Sheen, Emilio Estevez, Jamie Lee Curtis, Jeff Bridges, Jane Fonda, Drew Barrymore, Oprah Winfrey, Candice Bergen, Sting, Madonna, Karen Allen, Quincy Jones, and let's not forget Ruth Buzzi!

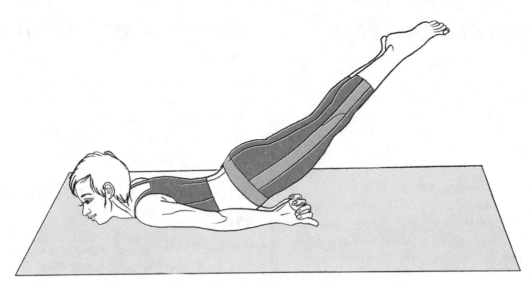

Locust pose.

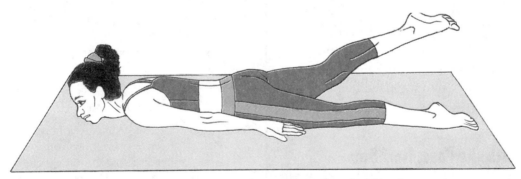

Single-Leg Locust pose is a great beginner's pose to build back strength.

Dhanurasana: Bow Pose

Dhanurasana (*DAH-noo-RAH-sah-nah*), or Bow pose, is a high-energy pose. Imagine your body is like an archer's bow ready to launch an arrow. This pose keeps your spine supple, tones your abdomen, massages your back muscles, strengthens your concentration, and decreases laziness.

When in Bow pose, be sure to grab your ankles, not your toes or feet. If you can't grab your ankles, simply bring your hands back as far as you can alongside your body. Keep your elbows straight, not bent, and don't lift your shoulders up to your ears—keep them pressed down. Open your chest, lengthen your torso, and breathe!

1. Lie on your stomach. Bring both arms behind you and bend both knees.

2. Grasp your ankles with your hands.

3. Pull your body so it lengthens like a bow and look up. Continue extending for two or three breaths.

Easing into the Pose: Half Bow

In Half Bow, the bow is strung one string at a time. When in Half Bow, be careful not to lean over to the side that is held straight. Balance both sides of your body, and be sure to breathe.

1. Begin on your stomach as with Bow pose, but extend your left arm straight over your head, palm down.

2. Bend your right knee and bring your right arm back toward your right ankle.

3. Push your stomach into the floor with your tailbone tipped toward the floor. Lift your head and chest. Keep your focus on your outstretched arm.

Easing into the Pose: Preparing for Full Bow

This preparatory pose might look easier than the full Bow pose, but don't be fooled. You need the same concentration as with Bow pose. This pose is a preparation for Bow pose, so hold it for only a few breaths on each side.

Continuing the Challenge: Rocking Bow

Rocking Bow is the full Bow plus! It aids digestion, relieves constipation, and tones the intestines.

In Bow pose, rock your body back and forth. Inhale as your body rocks back, exhale as you rock forward. Keep your arms straight. You can even add some rock-n-roll to this pose by doing it to your favorite song.

> **Wise Yogi Tells Us**
>
> Swami Vishnu Devananda says, "Om is a bow, the arrow is the Soul, Brahman [absolute bliss] is the arrow's goal."

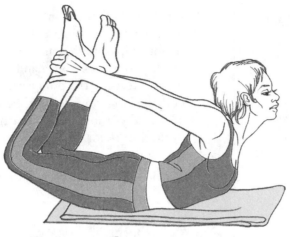

Bow pose.

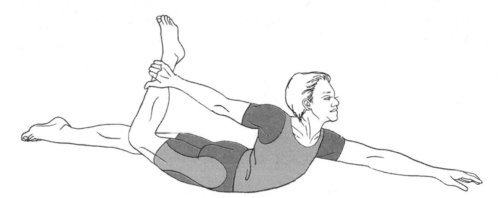

Half Bow pose.

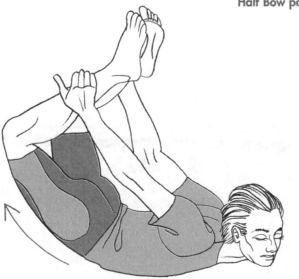

Rocking Bow pose.

Urdhvamukha Shvanasana: Upward Facing Dog

Urdhva means "upward," *mukha* means "mouth" or "face," and *shvan* means "dog." Urdhva-mukha shvanasana (*OORD-vah-MOOK-hah shvah-NAH-sahn-ah*) looks like a dog stretching upward. Upward Facing Dog is great for a stiff back. It strengthens the spine, alleviates back-aches, increases respiration and circulation (especially to the pelvic area), and strengthens the eyes.

1. Go into Cobra pose, then inhale deeper and straighten your arms, keeping your legs strong. (This takes the pressure off your back.)

2. Inhale and lift the front of your body off the floor as you look up. Continue to lift so your hips and legs are held just slightly off the floor, too. Your hands and the tops of your feet are the only parts of your body making contact with the floor in this advanced version. Let your arms do much of the work, not just your spine (as in Cobra pose).

3. Exhale as you come back down to the floor.

Ouch!

Be careful not to let your legs roll inward while in Upward Facing Dog. Lift your inner legs. If you feel off-balance, concentrate on centering your balance on your feet. Weak legs will cause your back to curve in and hurt. Keep them strong!

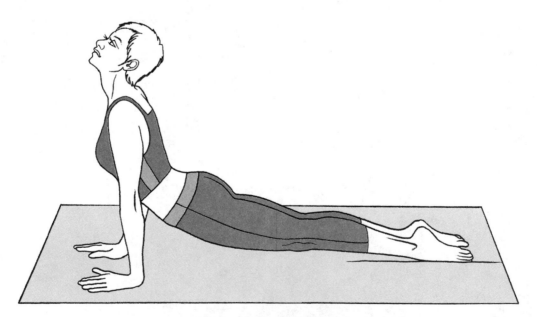

Upward Facing Dog pose.

Kapotasana: Pigeon Pose

Pigeon flows naturally from Upward Facing Dog. It opens the chest, hips, and throat and increases flexibility in the spine.

1. Begin in Downward Facing Dog pose.

2. Exhale and draw one leg forward. Place your foot in front of your hips, knee bent and pointing forward. Support yourself by resting your fingers on the ground on both sides of your hips. This might be far enough for most of us and is an excellent version of Pigeon pose. If you would like to take this pose further …

3. Inhale and bend the knee of the leg behind you as you reach back with your head toward your foot.

4. Eventually, work to the point where you can touch the crown of your head with the toes of the foot behind you. This is King Pigeon!

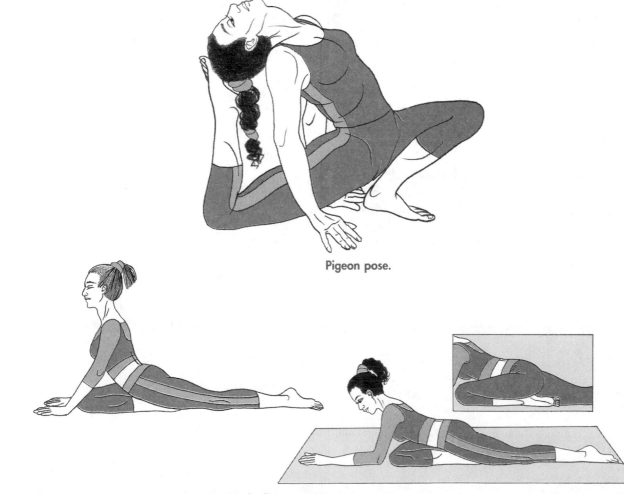

Pigeon pose.

Move gradually into Pigeon pose.

Matsyasana: Go Fish

Matsyasana (*mahtz-YAH-sah-nah*) fills the lungs with air, improving the yogi's ability to float in water. Fish pose energizes the parathyroid gland (which regulates calcium in your body), strengthens the abdomen, improves the voice by opening the fifth chakra (throat), and relieves mental tension.

1. Lie flat on your back with your feet to-gether and your knees straight.

2. Place your palms facing down under your tailbone with your thumbs touching.

3. Inhale, then lift your upper chest and arch your back, supporting your weight with your arms and elbows. Allow your head to tilt back.

4. Rest the top of your head lightly on the floor. Feel the strength of the lift in your arms and chest. Hold for three breaths, then exhale as you come down.

Easing into the Pose: Half Fish Pose

Start with Half Fish pose and work your way up to the full Fish. In the Half Fish pose, don't let your feet fall to the side. Keep your knees straight. Relax your head back and arch your back up high so that the top of your head eventually rests on the floor. Keep your elbows in, breathe regularly, and don't put your weight on your head. Let your elbows and arms support your weight.

If you have a stiff neck, jaw, or upper back, place a folded towel, blanket, or bolster-type pillow under your neck and gently look up and back to accustom your neck and head to this position.

Backbends make it easier to breathe deeply by opening up the chest and abdomen. The deep breathing gets more oxygen to the brain. As a result, you feel stimulated, refreshed, and energized. Combine backbends with forward bends to relax your spine. You may find you start craving backbends.

Continuing the Challenge: Full Fish Pose

This is like Half Fish pose, except your legs and feet are in the full Lotus position (see Chapter 9) and your hands hold your feet. If you cannot do the full Lotus, simply cross your legs. If you aren't in full Lotus position, you don't need to hold your feet. This variation further opens the pelvis and promotes energy flow through all your chakras.

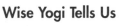

Wise Yogi Tells Us

Certain poses can help open certain chakras. To open a chakra, concentrate on the chakra while holding the pose. Feel the energy flowing through and from the target chakra. Feel the energy soar!

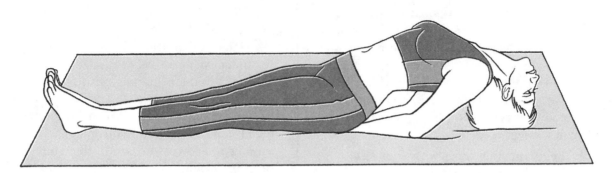

Half Fish pose.

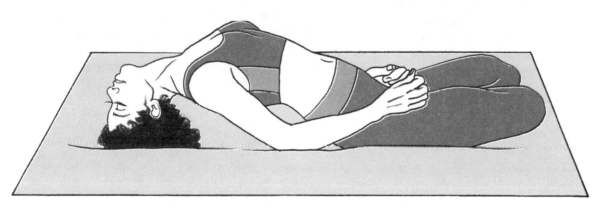

Full Fish pose.

Ustrasana: Camel

Ustra means "camel," and *ustrasana* (*oohs-TRAH-sah-nah*) imitates the body of a camel. This pose opens your shoulders and chest, stretches your abdomen, improves your digestion, and strengthens your rib muscles. This pose can also help sciatica, an inflammation in the nerve that runs from the hip down the back of the leg.

1. Begin on your knees with your feet behind you, legs and feet together or slightly apart.

2. Stretch your hips and thighs forward as you reach behind you with your arms. Extend your spine and lift upward as you lean back.

3. Let your body bend backward and your chin lift up. Look up. If you can't reach your heels, simply rest your hands on your buttocks. Take it gradually.

4. Take several deep breaths in the pose, then exhale as you release and come forward to the beginning position.

When practicing the Camel pose, pretend there is a wall in front of you and you are pressing your thighs toward it. Bend only as far backward as you can while keeping your neck properly supported by your neck muscles.

If this pose is too difficult, you can place a chair or a footstool behind you and use it to support your elbows or hands behind you. Remember not to let your head hang loosely, but to support it with your neck muscles as you look up.

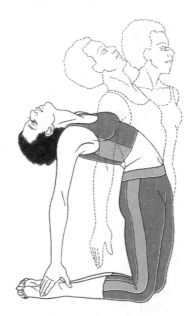

Camel pose.

Cakrasana: Doin' Wheelies!

Cakrasana (*chah-KRAH-sah-nah*) or Wheel pose makes your body strong and mobile, like a wheel. It stretches and strengthens the stomach, improves the concentration by bringing blood to the head, and gives greater control over the body.

1. Lie flat on your back with your knees bent, feet flat on the floor.

2. Bend your elbows toward the sky and bring your palms to the floor next to your ears, fingers facing your feet.

3. Lift your navel (think of lifting your third chakra, located behind your navel), and push your torso up into an arch using your arms and legs. Your head should be off the floor, and your arms and legs will be almost straight.

4. Hold for as long as is comfortable, then gently come back down.

Easing into the Pose: Modified Wheel Pose

If the full Wheel pose is too difficult, modify it by keeping your stomach flat and your elbows and knees bent, so you aren't pushing yourself all the way up. You can leave your head resting on the floor between your hands. In Wheel pose, your hips might feel too tight to extend sufficiently. If your shoulders are tight or your arms are weak, you might be unable to push yourself up into position.

Moving into Wheel pose.

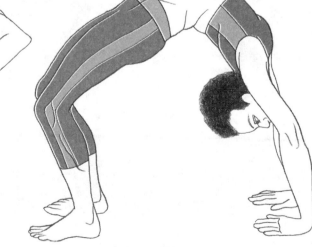

Wheel pose.

A Yoga Minute

The Sanskrit name for Wheel pose, cakrasana, is named after the chakras, or cakras, because it is the one pose that effectively stimulates all the chakras in your body. Chakras are often depicted as wheels, hence the name of the Wheel pose: cakrasana.

Continuing the Challenge

To get into Elbows to Ground pose, slowly lower your body down onto your elbows, your hands pointing toward your feet. Then, slowly raise one leg up. Don't attempt this pose unless your balance in Wheel pose is very secure and you have good flexibility.

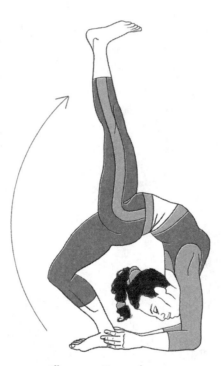

Elbows-to-Ground pose.

The Least You Need to Know

◆ Back-bending poses are important for increasing flexibility, as well as keeping various internal organs open and free.

◆ Open, toned organs result in open chakras and a free flow of energy throughout the body.

◆ Backbends are great for people who work at desks or computers all day; they correct that hunched-over posture.

◆ Backbends make it easier to breathe deeply and fully; they stimulate the body and get more oxygen to the brain.

◆ Backbends bring fuller laughs into our lives!

In This Chapter

◆ Gentle twists to realign your spine

◆ Inversions to invigorate

◆ Spinal twists to scintillate

◆ Modifications, challenges, and other tips to improve your yoga practice

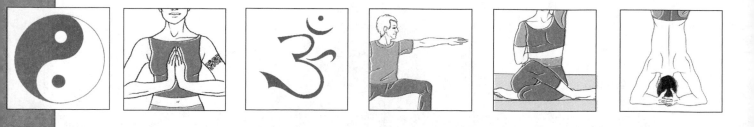

Chapter 8

Upside Down and All Around!

Twists are wonderful ways to clear out your system. They free and realign your spine so that every part of your body works better. Twists massage the internal organs and help the body force toxins out. Prana is allowed to enter the spine and energize it. For balance, always remember to do *both* sides of a spinal twist.

Inversions, on the other hand, can be described as the fountain of youth. They are amazing postures that balance all that standing and walking around right side up. Blood flows to the brain, gravity works the other way on every part of your body—after a good headstand, you'll feel almost like you've spent the day at a spa.

Maricyasana: Spinal Twist

Maricyasana (*MAH-rih-si-AH-sah-nah*) gives the spine a nice, lateral stretch, increasing spinal elasticity. The spinal twist also improves side-to-side mobility; decreases backaches and hip pain; contracts and tones the liver, spleen, and intestines; reduces abdominal size; improves the nervous system; prevents calcification at the base of the spine; frees the joints; and rouses your kundalini energy.

1. Sit on the floor with both legs out in front of you.

2. Bend your left leg over the outside of your right leg, then turn to the left.

3. Bend your right arm and place your right elbow on the outside of your left knee. Keep your shoulders down.

4. Lift your spine and twist, looking behind you as you push your chest forward (in the direction you are facing) to lengthen your spine.

5. Return to the starting position and repeat on the other side.

Ouch!

In Spinal Twist, don't overtwist your neck. Keep the twist the full length of your spine for full benefit. Keep the movement slow and deliberate, no matter how advanced you are. Keep your bent knee facing upward to support a steady twist of your spine. Count five breaths as you twist to look behind you, then five breaths to twist back to center.

Bound Knee Spinal Twist

This variation opens your hips as Spinal Twist does, but be sure to keep your back straight and shoulders down. And remember to enjoy

this pose. This is a more advanced twist, and if you aren't enjoying it, skip it for now and try a different spinal twist instead. If you can't quite connect your hands, just reach them toward each other. You'll get there eventually.

1. From a sitting position with your legs straight out in front of you, bend your left knee and bring your heel in, right up against your body.

2. Turn to your right, bringing your left shoulder around your left knee.

3. Bring your right arm behind your back and connect your hands.

Lying Down Spinal Twist

This variation tones the spine and strengthens the legs. It can also be quite relaxing as gravity helps you out.

1. Begin by lying down with your knees bent and your palms together in front of your chest, as if in prayer (namaste).

2. Straighten your arms toward the sky, and let your knees and outstretched arms drop (control the movement) to the right.

3. Lift your left arm and bring it up and over so it rests on your left side. Your arms are extended so your body makes a T. Gently turn your head and look at your left hand.

4. Breathe. Enjoy. Relax.

5. Turn your head back to the right, bring your left hand back to your right hand, then gently bring your knees back to center.

6. Repeat on the other side.

7. For an extra challenge, practice deep breathing while resting in Lying Down Spinal Twist. The twist adds resistance to the expansion of your lungs, strengthening all the muscles used for breathing.

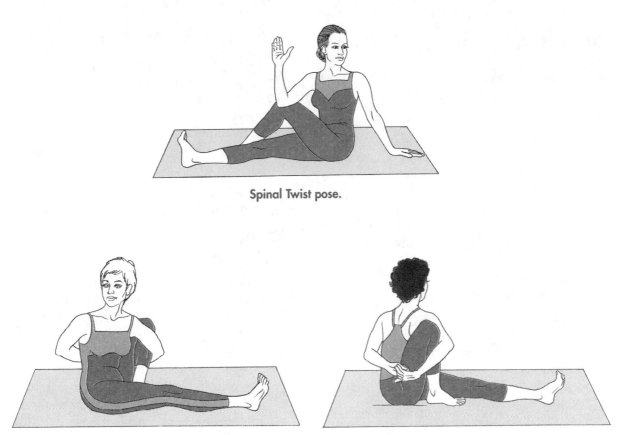

Spinal Twist pose.

Bound Knee Spinal Twist to the right and to the left.

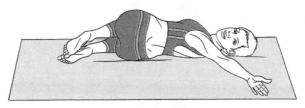

Lying Down Spinal Twist.

Setu Bandha Sarvangasana: Bridge Pose

Setu bandha sarvangasana (*SAY-too BAHN-dah SAHR-vahn-GAH-sah-nah*) is Bridge Pose. *Setu* means "bridge," and *sarvangasana* is composed of *sarva* ("all"), *anga* ("limb"), and of course, *asana* ("posture"). Setu bandha sarvangasana does indeed look like a bridge, and it strengthens the neck and back; tones the entire spine; builds supple wrists; and soothes the pituitary, thyroid, and adrenal glands with blood and other nutrients. Bridge pose helps intestinal function as well. This pose is a good preliminary to Shoulderstand.

1. Lie flat on the floor, with your knees bent and your feet flat on the floor about hip distance apart. Keep your hands to your sides.

2. Grab your ankles and bring them directly under your bent knees. Lift your hips, creating a bridge shape. Place your hands under your lower back for support, pointing your fingers in toward your spine. Keep your elbows next to your body. Your head, neck, and shoulders should stay on the floor.

3. Tighten your buttocks muscles to support your lifted torso. Make sure your knees are aligned with your ankles, that they face forward, and that they don't fall in or out as you hold the pose.

Easing into the Pose: Half Bridge

If Bridge pose is too difficult, start with Half Bridge pose. Clasp your hands under your body, drawing your elbows in so your arms are straight and resting on the floor underneath you. Concentrate on lifting your body as high as you can. This pose builds strength and flexibility to prepare your body for the full Bridge pose.

Continuing the Challenge: Extended Bridge

For an even greater strength challenge, try Extended Bridge pose. Walk your feet out, away from your body, until your legs are straight. Keep those abdominals lifted and buttocks muscles working—you don't want your bridge to sag! Extended Bridge is a very difficult pose that takes a lot of torso strength. Be kind to your back. If it hurts, bring your knees back to a bent position. Remember yoga's first principle? Ahimsa—nonviolence!

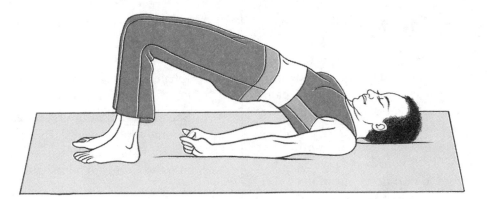

Half Bridge pose.

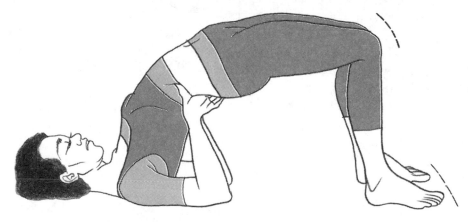

Bridge pose.

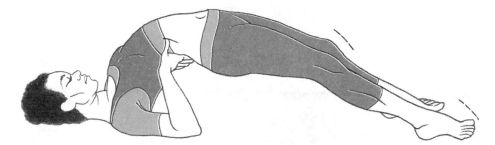

Extended Bridge pose.

Wallflower Stretch

Inversions can be a real challenge for some people who find it disconcerting to be upside down. To ease into inversions, or just to spend a really great 15 minutes after a hectic day, try Wallflower Stretch. Although not a classical yoga pose, this rejuvenating inversion takes very little effort but offers great benefits to your body, especially to tired legs and feet. Blood flows out of the lower extremities but the support of the wall makes this stretch so easy that anyone can do it, even those who have never tried a yoga pose before. All you need is a wall and possibly a folded blanket, towel, or small pillow. Wallflower Stretch also helps us see things in a whole new light. With our legs up the wall, our heads on the ground, and our arms and chests open to possibility, who knows what great inspiration could dawn!

1. Lie on the floor and scoot your hips up to a wall. Gently lift your legs and place them against the wall so your body forms a right angle with your legs up the wall and your torso on the floor. Keep your feet relaxed in a natural flexed position.

2. If it's more comfortable, place a folded blanket, towel, or small pillow under your head, neck, and/or hips.

3. Inhale and open your arms, bringing them beside your head, palms open and relaxed.

4. Spend about 15 minutes here, breathing naturally and relaxing. Do a quick body scan to search out areas of tension, and breathe into these areas to release the tension.

 A Yoga Minute

Wallflower Stretch is great for women who are suffering from the cramps of premenstrual syndrome. Although some yoga literature advises against inversions for menstruating women, this is okay because it doesn't invert your abdomen. It can also be healing for men with prostate concerns. Wallflower Stretch is conducive to inner reflection and a deep tranquility, in addition to a profound sense of relaxation—all of which can help alleviate emotional upheavals and physical discomforts.

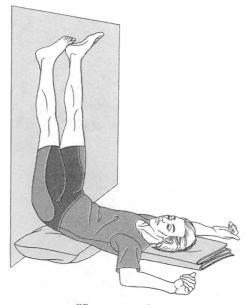

Wallflower Stretch pose.

Sarvangasana: Shoulderstand

Sarvangasana (*SAHR-vahn-GAH-sah-nah*) is a great inversion that stimulates the thyroid gland and the fifth chakra (throat). It reverses the pull of gravity on your internal organs and reduces the strain on your heart, because your heart doesn't have to work as hard to pump to the extremities when inverted. The Shoulderstand helps with varicose veins; purifies the blood; nourishes the brain, lungs, and heart; strengthens the eyesight; and helps clear the mind.

1. Lie flat on the floor, then bring both legs and hips up in the air. Lift up by contracting your abdominal and buttocks muscles. Although a little bit of a swing can help you get up there, let your muscles do most of the work.

2. Support your lower back with your hands so your upper arms are resting on the floor behind you, your elbows are bent, and your

hands rest on your back with your fingers facing inward, toward your spine.

3. Bring your shoulders away from your ears and push your feet toward the ceiling, almost as if you were hanging by your feet. Breathe! (You'll probably notice that breathing feels different upside down.)

Ouch!

To protect your neck, it is best to begin your exploration of Shoulderstand under the guidance of an instructor. Remember not to crunch your neck, and make sure not to twist it. Think of your neck lengthening as you hold the pose. Put a folded towel or blanket right at the tip of your shoulders to allow more room for your neck to stretch. And don't forget to breathe! Keep your elbows firmly grounded and keep your neck lengthened and your feet together.

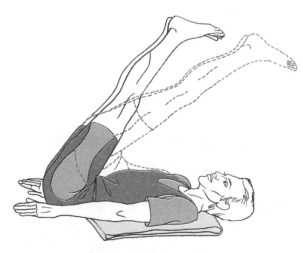

Moving into Shoulderstand pose.

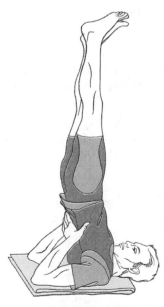

Shoulderstand pose.

Halasana: Plough Pose

Halasana (*hah-LAH-sah-nah*) looks like a plough, and *hala* means "plough." Plough pose folds the torso, compressing the internal organs and digestive system. The effect is to suffuse the internal organs and organ systems of the torso with energy, stimulating the stomach and digestive tract, alleviating constipation, and energizing the spleen, liver, gall bladder, and kidneys. Plough also stimulates the spine, strengthens the nervous system, improves circulation, releases neck tension, decreases insomnia, promotes mental relaxation, activates the third (throat) chakra, improves communication, and stimulates the heart.

1. Lie on your back with your knees bent, feet flat on the floor, and hands at your waist.

2. Inhale and raise your legs, hips, and buttocks off the ground into Shoulderstand. Steady yourself in Shoulderstand. After several breaths there, begin to slowly bring your legs backward, keeping your legs together and straight.

3. Exhale as you lower your feet to the floor behind your head. As soon as you start to feel undue strain in your back, hold your feet and don't bring them down any farther. Touch your legs to the ground only when they are straight and you feel no painful strain in your neck or back.

4. Clasp your hands under your body, facing away from your feet.

Easing into the Pose

In Plough pose, be sure to keep your knees straight. Don't twist your head or neck. Don't force your toes to the ground; let gravity do this slowly. If your toes seem like they aren't even close, try Plough pose with a chair or large pillow behind you so your feet can rest on something a little higher.

Continuing the Challenge: Hands-to-Feet

For an even greater challenge in Plough pose, try the Hands-to-Feet variation. This variation is identical to the first Plough, except that you stretch your arms along the ground until they touch your feet. This pose further opens and stretches the shoulders. Notice that this pose looks like an upside-down forward bend. In fact, you might begin to notice that many "different" poses are really the same, just gravitationally different. (Meditate on that for a while!)

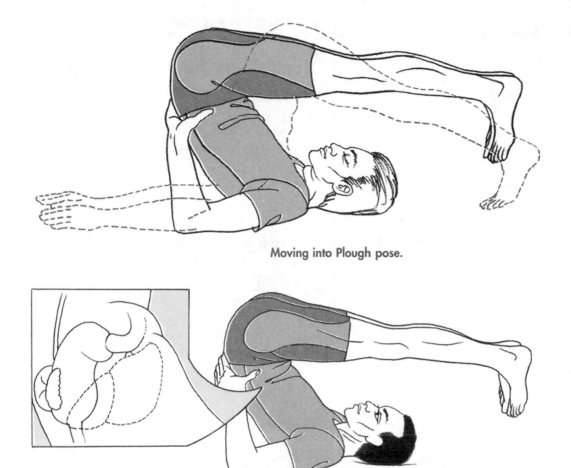

Moving into Plough pose.

Plough pose compresses the torso, stimulating the stomach and helping activate the digestive system. Plough pose also energizes the gallbladder, kidneys, and spleen.

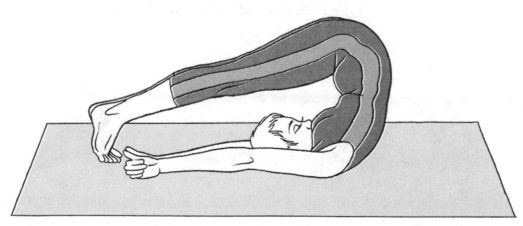

Hands-to-Feet pose.

Dolphin Stretch

Dolphin Stretch is an energizing and arm-strengthening movement that helps prepare the body for Headstand. This movement builds shoulder strength, aligns the upper back and shoulders, and helps with mental clarity and focus. It is an excellent movement for building upper-body strength, and can make not only Headstand but also Handstand and Downward Facing Dog feel more comfortable.

1. Begin on your hands and knees with your knees beneath your hips, your toes on the floor. Bring your elbows down to the floor, shoulder width apart. Clasp your hands together so your forearms form a V on the floor, keeping your elbows shoulder width apart.

2. Inhale and slowly straighten your legs, lifting your hips into the air. You can either keep your hands clasped or place them palms down. Drop your head down so the top of your forehead just lightly touches or hovers about an inch off the floor.

3. Slowly bring your heels down as far as possible. Don't worry if you can't put your foot flat on the floor; just feel a nice calf stretch.

4. Breathe steadily, then exhale as you lower your body and rock forward to bring your chin down to the floor to touch your hands.

5. Inhale as you come back up into Elbow Dog (Downward Facing Dog, but with your upper body resting on elbows and forearms instead of hands).

6. Exhale as you rock your body forward and touch your chin to your hands. Continue this movement back and forth, and imagine yourself a dolphin moving through the water.

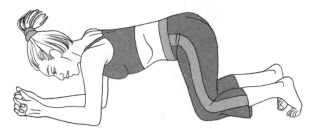

Begin the Dolphin Stretch from this position.

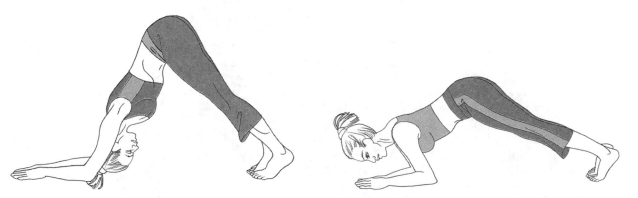

Dolphin Stretch movement. You may keep your hands clasped or stretch them out, as shown, as long as you feel stable and comfortable.

Shirshasana: Headstand

Shirshasana (*sher-SHAH-sahn-ah*) is probably one of the most famous yoga poses and is considered the king of the Hatha Yoga poses (Shoulderstand is queen). Headstand stimulates the whole system, improving circulation and strengthening the nervous system, emotions, and brain.

To make sure your body is ready, you must have sufficient arm, shoulder, neck, and stomach strength, plus be well versed in tadasana, Mountain pose, so you can balance your weight evenly while upside down. Most of the weight is in your arms in this pose. Your arms, shoulders, and even the stabilizing strength of a strong abdomen support your bodyweight. Your head is a balance point in the pose.

Ouch!

Heads aren't meant to bear your entire weight, and you could injure your neck if you put too much pressure on your head. Instead, your head is merely one of the minor supporting points in the supportive triangle you create with your arms.

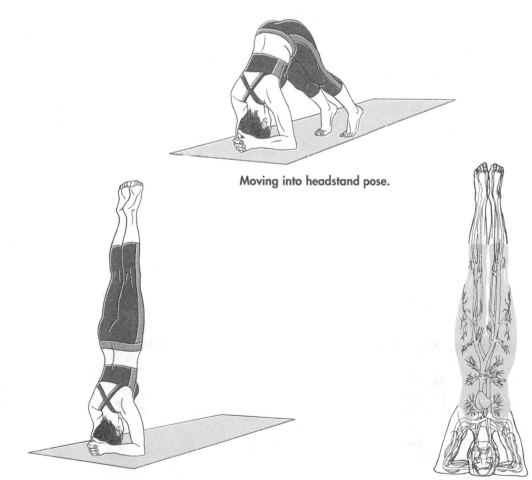

Moving into headstand pose.

Headstand pose.

In Headstand, gravity takes over, funneling blood back through your circulatory system, making the work much easier for your heart.

When first attempting Headstand, use a wall for support. The more comfortable and strong you become, the less you'll need the wall, until soon you'll be doing Headstands anytime, anywhere!

1. Get down on your hands and knees. Grab your left elbow with your right hand and your right elbow with your left hand.

2. Bring your elbows to the ground and release your hands. Keep your elbows shoulder distance apart for best support.

3. Interlace your fingers so your arms form a point, then cup the top of your head in your palms at the top of the point, as if your head were inside the apex of a triangle.

4. Slowly walk your feet in toward your body, straightening your back, then slowly raise your feet into the air.

5. Breathe! Try to stay balanced in Headstand for at least a few even breaths. Then come back down slowly. Remain with your head down for a few minutes before sitting up.

Ouch!

As wonderful a pose as Headstand is, it shouldn't be practiced under certain circumstances. If you have high blood pressure, heart problems, or are pregnant, do not attempt Headstand or any of the inverted poses. You might still be able to do inversions with no problem, but talk to your yoga-friendly doctor first.

Easing into the Pose

Balancing in a headstand isn't just a matter of lifting your feet up and hanging out for a while. As your proficiency increases, so does your awareness. Your entire body will be making minor adjustments, tiny movements, little shifts here and there—along your arms, shoulders, hands, neck, back, and legs—to keep you balanced. Notice how your body tries to compensate to keep you balanced. Your body knows. Learn from it!

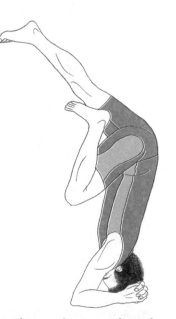

This poorly executed Headstand is out of alignment.

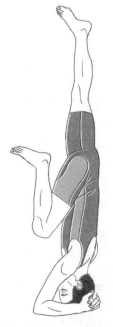

In a correct Headstand, your hips and torso align with your long straight neck, head, and shoulders.

Continuing the Challenge: Variations

Experienced Headstanders can try other changes in leg position, such as bending your knees, moving your legs apart, bringing the soles of your feet together, or the lovely and symmetrical Lotus Headstand, padma shirshasana (*PAHD-mah sher-SHAH-sah-nah*). While in Headstand, move your legs slowly and keep control over your balance. For Lotus Headstand, you must be able to bring your feet into the full Lotus position without the help of your hands.

For any Headstand variation, be very careful when shifting your legs because any quick shifts in bodyweight, especially unevenly on one side, could cause muscle strain or vertebral damage to your neck, upper back, or lower back. Always move slowly to maintain your balance and keep your Headstand stabilized so your hips and torso remain in a straight line over your head. Because Headstand variations are advanced poses, consult a qualified teacher for personal guidance.

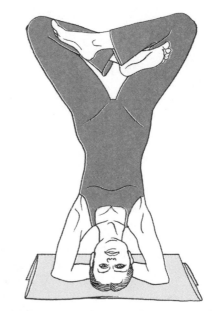

The Lotus Headstand—a challenging Headstand variation.

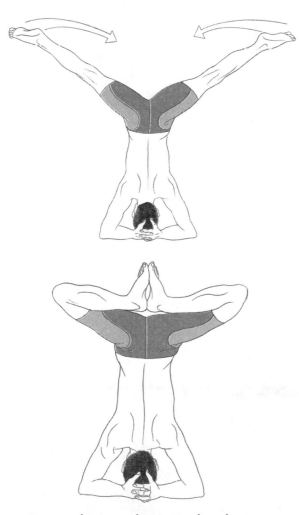

Once you become adept in Headstand, you may vary your pose by slowly moving your legs into different positions while maintaining centered stability.

Vrichikasana: Scorpion Pose

Scorpion pose mimics the unusual form and curve of the scorpion. This pose is extremely challenging and takes upper body strength, balance, concentration, and confidence. You should feel very comfortable with Headstand and be strong enough to hold it comfortably for about five minutes before attempting this pose.

1. Start in Headstand. Slowly release your hands and bring them apart, pressing your palms against the floor.

2. Slowly lift your head slightly off the ground and bend your knees, balancing so the curve of your torso offsets the weight of your lower legs.

3. If you feel very comfortable, try bending your knees so your toes touch your forehead, or straightening your legs all the way up.

Scorpion pose takes great physical and mental strength, but in turn, it imbues the bodymind with a great sense of inner strength and balance.

Adho Mukha Vrksasana: Handstand

Adho mukha vrksasana (*AHD-hoh MOOK-hah vrik-SHA-sah-nah*) requires great arm strength to do properly. Practice Downward Facing Dog (see Chapter 11) to develop your arms and prepare your body for Handstand.

Handstand gives you tremendous energy. It strengthens your arms and shoulders, plus gives you all the blood-cleansing effects of inversions. If trying this pose scares you, work with a partner who can spot you. The Handstand, however, requires a lot of combined abdominal and upper-body strength. If you're not strong enough, continue building strength through Dolphin, Headstand, and Downward Facing Dog.

1. Do Downward Facing Dog (see Chapter 11) in front of a wall. Place your hands on the floor, shoulder width apart, and about three to five inches from the wall. Slowly walk your legs in toward the wall.

2. Exhale and lift one leg straight up. Follow quickly with the other in a gentle kicking-up motion. Keep your arms and legs straight and firm. Push your shoulders away from the floor, and rest your outstretched legs lightly against the wall.

3. Hold the pose for as long as is comfortable. Breathe! Exhale as you come down.

Know Your Sanskrit

Adho mukha means "face down," and *vrksa* means "tree," so Handstand, **adho mukha vrksasana,** is Tree pose turned upside down.

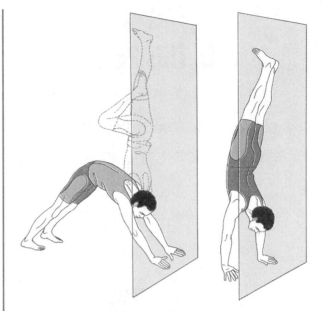

Moving from Downward Facing Dog pose into Handstand pose.

The Least You Need to Know

◆ Spinal twists gently massage internal organs, strengthen the spine, and purify your system.

◆ Inversions—the Bridge, Shoulderstand, Plough, Headstand, and Handstand—are yoga's fountain of youth: they keep you young!

◆ Inversions send blood to the brain—that's brain power!

◆ Avoid inversions if you have high blood pressure, heart problems, or are pregnant.

In This Part

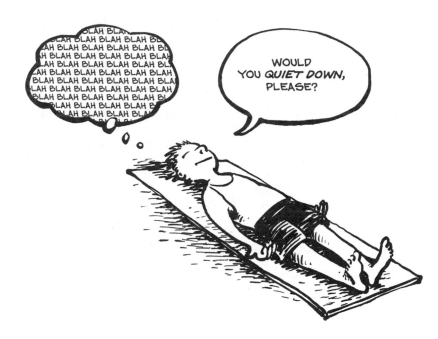

Part 3

Calm: Postures to Quiet the Body and Mind

The poses (asanas) in Part 3 balance out the poses in Part 2. While the first series of asanas was energizing, these asanas calm and quiet the body and mind. First, we'll try some sitting poses, which center you in your body and create a tranquil mind. Poses such as the Lotus are prime for meditation, so we'll introduce you to other meditation techniques as well, including mudras and mantras.

Next, we'll tell you how to infuse your body with life-force energy through the yoga breathing exercises called pranayama. Then, we'll show you how forward-bending poses help you focus inward. Finally, we'll devote a chapter to the most important of all the poses: shavasana, or Corpse pose, which cultivates stillness.

In This Chapter

- ◆ Poses for confidence: Staff, Butterfly, Hero
- ◆ Cow pose: one sacred posture
- ◆ Special poses for meditation: Easy and Kneeling
- ◆ Finally, Lotus pose!

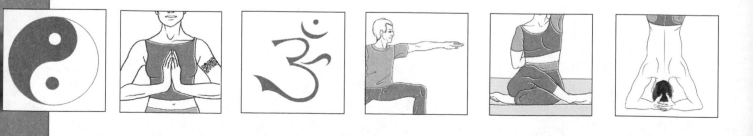

Chapter 9

Are You Sitting Down?

Many of yoga's sitting poses are ideal for meditating, while others are more challenging. Sitting poses such as Staff, Butterfly, Hero, and Cow keep your hips and legs flexible.

While you can meditate in just about any position, the meditative poses such as Easy pose, Kneeling pose, and Lotus pose arrange your body in a way that optimizes meditation. Your spine is aligned so energy can flow freely, and your body is relaxed and comfortable. You can enhance a meditative position with mudras, hand positions that channel energy back through the fingers into the spinal column's chakras, directing and rebalancing prana in the body.

So roll out your yoga mat, and let's get started!

Dandasana: Staff Pose

Staff pose can help you internalize a feeling of confidence, increase your concentration, and clarify your focus. Think for a moment about what a staff symbolizes. It can be a walking stick that you use for support, so it symbolizes strength. It also can represent authority, the person in charge. Also think "staff of life." In yoga, the staff represents *sushumna*, or the central channel of power.

Dandasana (*dahn-DAH-sah-nah*) is also great for your alignment. As you hold this pose, concentrate on your upper body becoming straight and powerful as a staff.

1. Sit on the floor with your feet straight out in front of you. Keep your palms flat alongside your hips with your fingers pointing toward your feet. Keep your knees and toes together, your heels pushed out, and your toes relaxed. Keep your shoulders down and your chest open.

2. Push your palms lightly down against the ground to create space in your spine. Lengthen the top and bottom of your body. Center your weight over your hips. Breathe.

3. If your palms do not touch the ground, place blocks or books under them for support. If your wrists hurt, make them into fists and rest upon the fists. A well-qualified yoga teacher can adjust any pose for your particular body needs.

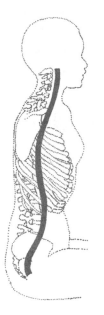

The proper alignment of your spine in Staff pose.

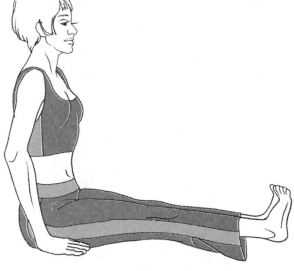

Staff pose.

Baddha Konasana: Butterfly Pose

Literally translated as "bound angle pose," this pose imitates a butterfly resting its wings on a lotus blossom. When holding baddha konasana (*BAH-dah koh-NAH-sah-nah*), imagine the delicate beauty of this image of the butterfly. Butterfly pose opens your hips and second chakra (see Appendix B) and loosens your knees and ankles.

If you are flexible, this pose may come easily to you. If not, you may want to place a pillow or blanket under each knee.

1. Sitting on the floor, bring the soles of your feet together, drawing them toward your body. Keep your back straight.

2. Open your chest and press your knees toward the ground as far as they will go. Don't bounce your legs up and down. Instead, allow gravity to gently release your hip joints.

3. Tilt your lower back inward to align the spine. Don't let your upper back hunch over. Keep your chin parallel to the floor.

4. As your hips loosen, you will eventually be able to bow forward with a flat back.

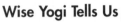

Wise Yogi Tells Us

While practicing Butterfly pose, keep your entire back straight. If you tend to round your upper back as you pull your feet in, place your feet farther from your body; hold on to your shins or thighs if you can't reach your feet. Concentrate on the image of the butterfly.

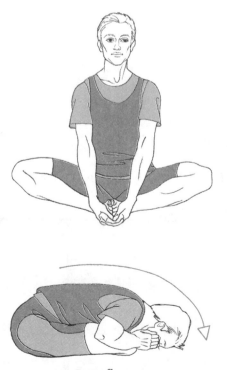

Butterfly pose.

Virasana: Be a Hero!

Hero pose refreshes your legs, stretches your knees, and balances your first chakra, located at the base of your spine (see Appendix B). Virasana (*vir-AH-sah-nah*) also teaches you to expand your breathing space even while sitting. Imagine lifting from the top of your head and anchoring your hips to the floor. Let your breath expand everything in between. If your knees are delicate, sit on a folded blanket, firm pillow, or block to lessen the stretch on the muscles of the knees.

1. Breathe deeply, filling your diaphragm.

2. Start by sitting back on a book, gradually separating your feet until you are fully sitting on the book between your legs. Find an old phone book, and each day rip out one page. Slowly your leg muscles will lengthen and you will work your way to the floor.

3. Keep your knees from buckling in, and slightly tilt your tailbone under, which lengthens the spine.

4. Pull your calf muscles out and away from your leg bones, preventing your knees from buckling in.

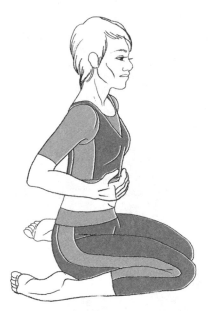

Feel your breath while sitting in Hero pose.

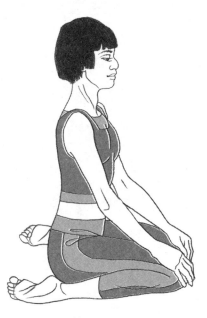

Hero pose.

Gomukhasana: Cow Pose

In India the cow is considered the most sacred of animals, so this pose is meant to enhance a feeling of openness and giving. It also stimulates the nerves at the base of your spine, aids in longevity as it keeps your lower vertebrae from calcifying, opens your shoulders and chest, activates your first and second chakras, and helps raise kundalini energy. In the word *gomukhasana* (*goh-moo-KHA-sah-nah*), *go* means "cow" and *mukha*, means "mouth" or "face."

1. Sit with your legs in front of you, then bring one knee on top of the other. Draw your heels toward your body in this cross-legged position.
2. Point one elbow toward the sky, with your palm facing your back behind you. Point your other elbow toward the ground, with your palm facing out behind you. Bring your hands toward each other, clasping them if you can for an invigorating shoulder stretch.

Easing into the Pose: A Yoga Strap

Don't be frustrated if your hands can't grasp each other, and don't force it. You don't want to pull a muscle! You'll get there eventually. Some people have less flexibility in their shoulders. If your hands don't touch in Cow pose, you can modify the pose by using a towel or yoga strap to get the same stretch and the same benefits.

Easing into the Pose: Cradle Rock

Cradle Rock is a gentle and relaxing movement that opens the hips in preparation for seated poses. Coming out of Cow pose, inhale and stretch your legs in front of you. Exhale as you bend one knee and grasp your ankle and calf with your hands. Gently rock your leg and calf in your arms, letting your hip joint release and relax. Repeat with the other leg.

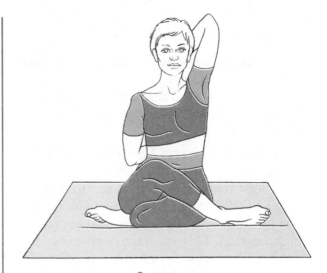

Cow pose.

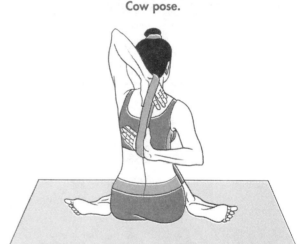

Bring your hands to touch in Cow pose. If you can't quite reach, use a strap or towel to feel the same stretch.

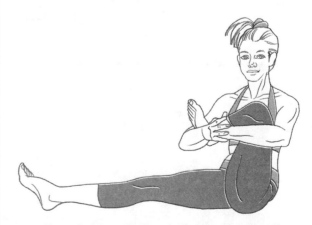

Cradle Rock opens the hips with a gentle, nurturing rock.

Sukhasana: Easy Pose

Sukhasana (*soo-KAH-sah-nah*) is a great meditation pose for beginners. *Sukha* means "joy," and this pose feels so good that it fills you with joy! Sukhasana facilitates pranayama, quiets the mind, and stills the body.

Sit in a simple crossed-leg position, with either leg on top. Try to sit more often with the leg that is least comfortable on top, to balance your body. Rest your hands on your knees and breathe. Don't be concerned if your knees do not yet rest on the ground. This will come in time as your hips open. If your back starts to arch, put a pillow under your tailbone to align your spine.

Vajrasana: Kneeling Pose

Vajrasana (*vahj-RAH-sah-nah*) is also called the Zen pose, because this is the meditation pose used by Zen Buddhist monks. *Vajra* means "thunderbolt" or "diamond." Vajrasana aids circulation to the feet, lifts the spinal column, and relieves pressure on the diaphragm. Sit back on your heels, keeping your heels and knees together. Keeping your spine straight, place your hands on your knees. If your knees hurt, go back to Easy pose. If they don't hurt, enjoy *this* pose.

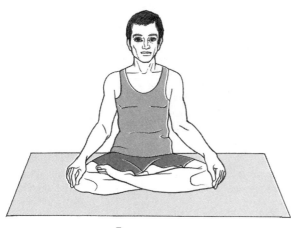

Easy pose.

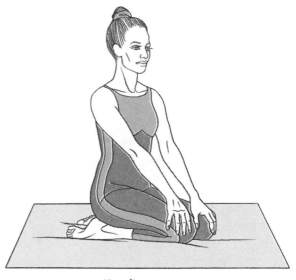

Kneeling pose.

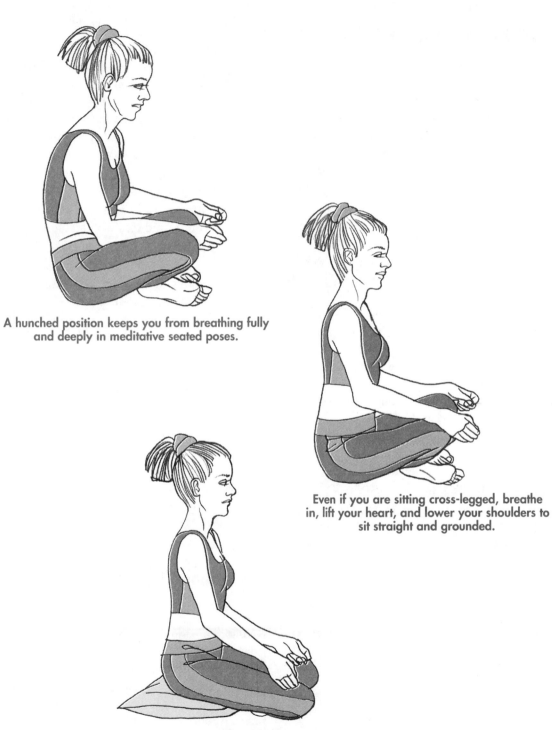

A hunched position keeps you from breathing fully
and deeply in meditative seated poses.

Even if you are sitting cross-legged, breathe
in, lift your heart, and lower your shoulders to
sit straight and grounded.

If you need more support, place a small pillow
under your buttocks; your knees will touch
the floor.

Padmasana: Lotus Pose

At last, the venerable Lotus pose! You've heard about it, maybe you've seen it, and perhaps you've even tried it. Padmasana (*pahd-MAH-sah-nah*) represents a lotus flower open to the light (*padma* means "lotus"). It keeps the spine from sagging and keeps you comfortable in meditation for longer periods of time than other positions. The Lotus position keeps your chest open, gives your diaphragm lots of room, and opens your fourth chakra, located behind your heart (see Appendix B).

The symbolism of the lotus flower is essential to yoga. The lotus flower is a beautiful circle of petals that floats on a lake or pond. The lotus roots, however, are deep in the mud. The mud provides the nutrients to help the lotus grow and achieve its beauty. To yogis, the lotus represents human life. Our lives are submerged in "mud"—rooted in the material world, in striving and grasping, in worry and pain. Yet we can use these challenges the way the lotus root absorbs nutrients from the mud—sending up a shoot that rises to the top of the murky lake and blooms on the surface in perfect beauty.

It's easy to be so concerned with trying to achieve Lotus pose that you forget the point of being in the pose: to be comfortable in your body and free your mind from distractions or worries. True meditation is joyful.

Ouch!

If your ankles, hips, or knees begin to hurt, return to Easy pose. Lotus pose requires strong ankles and open hips. Practice yoga's standing postures to build ankle and hip strength, then come back to Lotus pose when you're stronger.

1. Sit on the floor and breathe deeply.
2. Place your left ankle on top of your right thigh so the sole of your foot faces upward. Then move your right ankle to the top of your left thigh so the sole of your other foot faces upward. (It's good to do this the other way around, too, switching the foot that is on top.)
3. Shift a little to center your weight on your hip bones, then place your hands, palms up or down, on your knees. This pose should feel very stable.
4. Ideally, your body will form a tripod, with both knees and your body touching the ground. If you can't get your knees down toward the ground, you can sit on a cushion or pillow. This can also make the pose easier for people with less-flexible hips.

Easing into the Pose: Neck Stretch

This stretch helps tone the muscles in the neck that connect to the collarbone, balancing our neck muscles. Remember, Hatha Yoga is about balance! In Lotus or any relaxed seated pose, inhale and gently tip your head back slightly, pulling down gently on the muscles above your collarbone with your fingertips. Breathe and relax in this position for several moments.

Continuing the Challenge: Bound Lotus Pose

Baddha padmasana, or Bound Lotus pose, is the same as the Lotus, except that your right arm goes behind your back and holds your right foot, while your left arm goes behind your back and holds your left foot. This pose is even more stable and symmetrical than Lotus pose. Whichever arm crosses on top, go the opposite way next time. Baddha padmasana

(*BAH-dah pahd-MAH-sah-nah*) deepens all the benefits of Lotus pose, and you'll be able to breathe more deeply. Butterfly pose (described earlier in this chapter) is an excellent warmup for the hip flexibility needed for stability in Lotus and Bound Lotus poses.

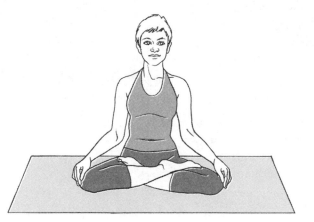

Lotus pose.

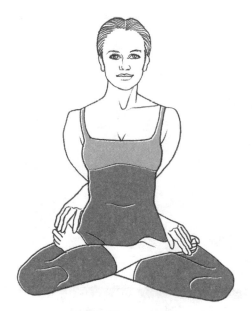

Bound Lotus pose.

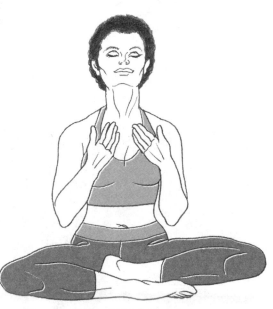

Seated Neck Stretch.

Continuing the Challenge: Lion in Lotus Pose

The Lion pose is a fun pose for kids as well as adults, but Lion pose is more than just fun. It gives all the facial muscles—from the tip of your tongue to the top of your forehead—a fantastic stretch.

1. Relax into Lotus pose. Inhale.

2. Exhale as you tip forward on your knees, placing your hands on the floor, fingers spread out, about two feet in front of your knees, shoulder width apart. Keep your legs in Lotus pose.

3. Inhale deeply, then as you exhale, open your mouth and eyes as wide as you can. Stick out your tongue as far as you can. Raise your eyebrows. Open your face as completely as you can.

4. Relax your face as you inhale. Repeat again on the exhale.

5. Rock back into Lotus pose and breathe normally for a few moments, relaxing the muscles of your face.

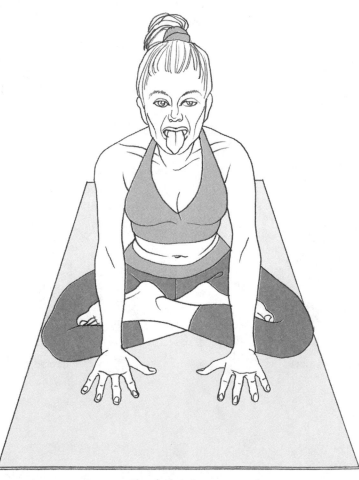

Lion in Lotus pose.

Continuing the Challenge: Tolasana, Scales Pose

Scales pose builds strength in the arms, shoulders, wrists, and hands. It also strengthens the abdominal muscles. You can do this pose while sitting in Easy pose if Lotus pose isn't comfortable for you yet. Make sure to contract your abdominal muscles as you lift, to help bring your legs and hips off the ground.

1. Sit in Lotus pose with your palms pressed firmly on the ground on both sides of your hips.

2. Exhale as you energize your arms and contract your abdominal muscles. Push down on the floor, lifting your feet and hips slightly off the ground. Hold as long as you can.

3. Repeat with your legs crossed the opposite way.

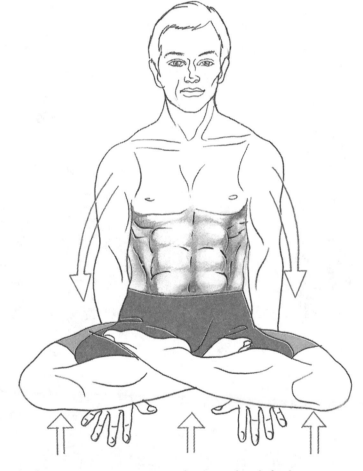

Scales pose. You may want to place your hands farther apart to hold steady in this pose, and that's okay!

Padandgushtasana: Big Toe Pose

Big Toe Pose, or padandgushtasana (*pah-dahnd-gush-TAH-sah-nah*) is a challenging balance pose that develops and strengthens your knees and ankles. It also promotes overall balance, stability, and confidence.

1. Begin standing in Prayer pose. Squat down with the weight balanced on the balls of your feet and your toes.

2. Pick a point of focus in front of you, and keep your eyes centered there for balance.

3. Once you have mastered this, try squatting down and then cross one foot up onto your other thigh. Let your top knee rest out to the side. Balance in this position for several steady breaths.

4. To come out of the pose, simply uncross your legs, sit down, and stretch your legs out.

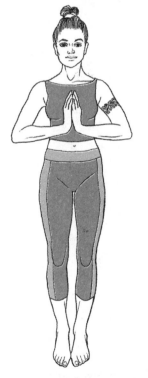

Start in Prayer pose.

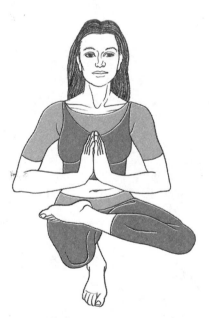

Squat into Big Toe pose.

Mudra Magic

Mudras refer to a variety of yoga practices that aren't poses exactly, but various techniques for sealing life-force energy inside the body. These techniques get pretty esoteric and can involve complex rituals, chanting, meditation, and some practices we Westerners might find unfamiliar.

The word *mudra*, however, is more commonly used today to refer to specific hand gestures used during meditation and pranayama to seal the fingers. Prana can escape out of the fingertips as it circulates through the body during meditation and pranayama exercises, and hand mudras bring the fingertips together in various ways for different, subtle effects. Hand mudras, in essence, create a prana circuit. The energy moves back around and into the body again.

Know Your Sanskrit

Mudra means "seal" in Sanskrit. A mudra is a hand position or gesture that seals life force energy at points in the body. By using a mudra, you create a closed, self-replenishing circuit of prana in your body.

Namaste Mudra: A Little Respect

Namaste mudra, or the respect gesture, puts the palms together in prayerlike fashion to honor the inner light in all of us. Place your palms together and extend your fingers upward, as if you are praying. Hold your hands to your heart.

Aum Mudra: Simply Divine

Aum mudra, or the divinity gesture, invokes divine balance. Open your palms, and with each hand, bring the tip of your thumb to the tip of your index finger to form a complete circle, which represents the complete cycle and ultimate harmony of divinity.

Jnana Mudra: Be a Wise Soul

Jnana (*GAH-nah*) mudra, or the wisdom gesture, produces wisdom. Rest your hands, palms up, on your knees, and touch each index finger to the middle of each thumb. The wisdom gesture promotes harmonious inward expression and openness to life's beauty. This mudra produces wisdom and encourages the ego to realize that relinquishment brings wisdom. This mudra is often practiced during meditation.

Buddhi Mudra: How Enlightening!

Buddhi mudra, or enlightenment gesture, is often associated with the Buddha and is ideal for centering and calming. Bring your thumb and index finger together, tip to tip, as in the Aum mudra. Then bring the back of your hands together, knuckles touching, and rest your hands against your lower abdomen at your second chakra (see Appendix B), the chakra that rules passion, creativity, sexuality, and creation of life. This mudra represents divinity and the oneness of self and also the joining of all energies. It quiets the mind, stills action, and enlightens the self to its inner divinity. Try this mudra when you are feeling tense or rushed.

Continuing the Challenge: Seeing the Light

Trataka (*trah-TAH-kah*) cleanses the eyes by focusing them on a candle flame until they start to water. Although you can do this eye exercise in any sitting position, Lotus pose makes for a strong and stable sitting position. Trataka is said to strengthen the eyes and, in some cases, induce clairvoyance. Trataka is a meditation technique with the candle flame as the point of focus.

Seated in Lotus pose, place a lighted candle a few feet in front of you at eye level. Choose a mudra and sit comfortably in meditative pose. Gaze at the flame. (Remember, don't get too close!) Make sure the candle flame is steady. It's important to eliminate drafts from the room. After a few minutes of gazing steadily at the flame, close your eyes. You will still be able to hold the image of the flame in your mind. Hold on to it as long as you can. If your eyes become irritated, rinse them in cold water and hold your gaze for a shorter time the next time around.

Mudras for Meditation

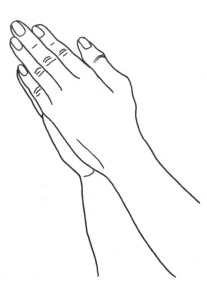

Namaste mudra.

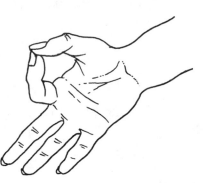

Aum mudra.

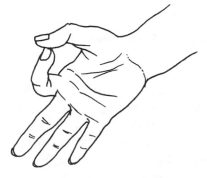

Jnana mudra.

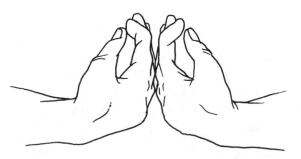

Buddhi mudra.

Mantras: Beyond Aum

If chanting seems a little too "out there" for you, bear with us. Once you understand what chanting is all about, you might just want to give it a try.

A *mantra* is a sound or sounds that resonate in the body and evoke certain energies. Mantras help stimulate the chakras by soothing your mind and awakening your senses. Herbert Benson, M.D., president and founder of the Mind/Body Medical Institute at Harvard Medical School, conducted many studies that showed how simple meditation including the repetition of a *mantra* (any word, sound, even a short prayer) induced a profound relaxation effect on the body. In his landmark book, *The Relaxation Response* (see Appendix D), Benson revealed the remarkable healing effects of this relaxation response. Yogis found the use of mantra (thought expressed as sound) effective thousands of years ago for inducing deeper states of consciousness.

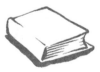

Know Your Sanskrit

A **mantra** is a sacred sound used in meditation as the object of focus, meant to resonate within the body and awaken the chakras. The word *mantra* is a composite of two Sanskrit root words. The first word, *man*, means "continual or constant thinking." The second word, *tra*, means "to be free." Mantra is a process by which you free yourself from worries or doubts, but not from consciousness.

Aum (also spelled Om) is a common mantra because it's designed to invoke a universal perspective: you see your bodymind in relation to its place in the big picture. In Sanskrit, Aum is spelled in three symbols that approximate the letters A-U-M, meant to invoke the resonating sound of this mantra.

Each letter is a sacred symbol:

◆ A represents the self in the material world.

◆ U represents the psychic realm.

◆ M represents indwelling spiritual light.

Chanting Aum unifies your perceptions so you can sense yourself as an integral part of the universe. Gradually, the chant helps you shed everything that separates you from the universe—all your negativity, illusions, and misperceptions of yourself and the world.

Aum Shanti Shanti Shanti is a great beginning mantra to try. *Shanti* means "peace," and when repeated three times, it balances the bodymindspirit.

The Least You Need to Know

◆ Sitting postures strengthen and increase flexibility in your hips and legs.

◆ Mudras are hand positions that enhance meditation by rechanneling energy that emanates from the fingers back into the body where it can stimulate the chakras.

◆ Meditate only in a posture that is perfectly comfortable. Some suggestions: Easy, Kneeling, and Lotus.

◆ Lotus pose can be a stabilizing base for many other yoga poses.

◆ Mantras are sounds, words, or phrases meant to resonate within the body.

In This Chapter

- ◆ The universal energy of prana
- ◆ How prana makes you feel better
- ◆ How to sit for optimal pranayama
- ◆ Some great pranayama techniques

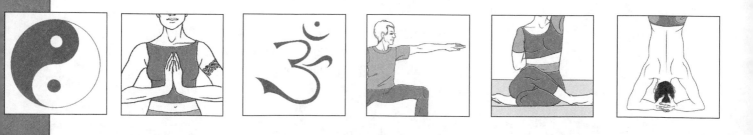

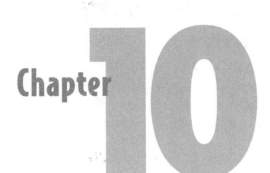

Chapter 10

Controlling the Power of Breath

Your breath and your mind have an intimate relationship. What your brain perceives, your breath mirrors and your body experiences. Imagine harnessing this power! Just as the mind influences the breath and body, the breath can influence the mind. Controlling the power of breath is the technique of pranayama, an integral part of Hatha Yoga.

The more prana, or life force energy, you bring into your body, the better your body and your mind will work, and the better you'll feel. Prana gives you instant energy and supports long-term good health. It is the ultimate feel-good medicine and a powerful preventive health-care tool.

So how do you develop prana inside you? By learning pranayama, or yoga breathing techniques.

Prana, the Universal Life Force

The deeper the breath, the deeper the life force. In Chapter 5, we described prana as the life force or energy that exists everywhere and is manifested in each of us through the breath, but prana isn't exactly the same thing as breath or oxygen. Prana exists in all living things. It doesn't have consciousness—it's pure energy. Every cell in your body is controlled by prana. Prana animates all matter.

Get in touch with the breath and the way prana infuses your body. Picturing the physiology (Western style!) of your thoracic cavity (the cavity containing your lungs and heart) might help you visualize what's happening as you breathe during pranayama. This is the area of your body that houses the diaphragm, that powerful, plate-shaped muscle that contracts and expands as you breathe. Inhale and imagine your diaphragm moving down in your body to expand the space in your lungs and rib cage. Exhale and imagine your diaphragm pushing up to guide the air out of your lungs.

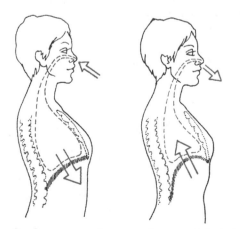

The diaphragm muscle moves down on inhalation and up on exhalation. Take a deep breath and feel the muscle in motion.

> **Wise Yogi Tells Us**
>
> According to wise yogis, the length of life is a matter of the number of breaths, not the number of years. Breath is so important to an accomplished yogi that he or she can get almost all necessary energy from the air. Sleeping? Eating? These are but minor concerns compared to the breath! That's why yogis have been known to sleep for just a few hours a night. All their energy is replenished through pranayama instead—the yogi's beauty sleep!

You can practice breathing exercises just about anywhere, but they'll be more productive if you practice them in certain positions. We encourage you to use one of the seated meditative poses from Chapter 9, such as Lotus pose. Or, practice breathing while lying in Corpse pose (see Chapter 12) or a variation of Corpse pose such as that shown in the illustration.

Just like anything else, breath control and capacity increase with practice. There is a practice called *kevali kumbhaka* (*kay-VAH-lee koom-BAH-kah*), in which you practice holding your breath. Don't make yourself dizzy, though, and don't hold your breath until you faint. Just hold your breath until you feel like you need to let it go again. The more you practice this technique, the longer you'll be able to hold your breath, which increases your lung capacity and makes your breathing more efficient.

Pranayama isn't difficult, but it takes concentration. There are many exercises to try, and following are a few. Experiment with each and consider incorporating a few of them into your yoga workout, between poses, before or after your workout, or whenever you need instant energy or calming.

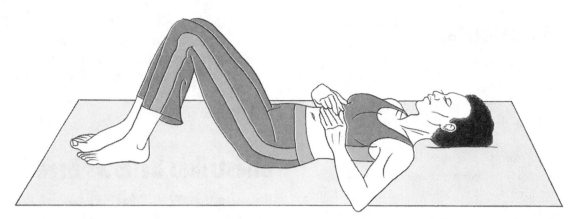

Lie on your back and place your hands over your lower ribs to feel the breath flowing in and out of your body.

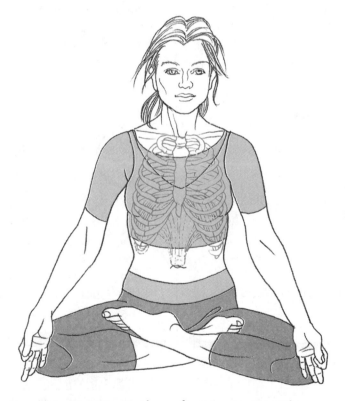

Lotus pose is a good pose for pranayama practice.

Om Exhalation

This technique extends the breath, softens it, and makes quieting the mind easier.

1. Inhale deeply, imagining your breath is moving all the way to the root of your spine.

2. Open your lips and begin to make the Aum sound while exhaling slowly: *Auuuuuuuuummmmmmmmm*, spending approximately 10 seconds on the "au" sound and about 5 seconds on the mmm sound. Count with your fingers. Keep the sound steady. Increase or decrease the seconds depending on the strength and steadiness of your sound.

3. Feel as if your entire being is enveloped in the sound. Let it surround and fill you.

4. Repeat several times.

Ujjayi: Drawing Breath

The *ujjayi* (oo-JAH-yee) technique aids in recalling and working with your dreams. It is also cooling to the head, aids digestion, soothes nerves, and tones the body. This breathing exercise produces sound in the throat with the inhalation.

Know Your Sanskrit

Jaya means "success on the spiritual path," and *ujjayi* means "one who is victorious." **Ujjayi** breath is a very empowering technique to add to your yoga practice.

1. Inhale slowly, keeping your lips closed and closing off the glottis, the opening between the vocal chords. Make a soft, humming sound: *hahhhhhhh*. Think Darth Vader breathing.

2. Imagine you are inhaling all the way to your heart. The upper portions of your lungs are full. You should feel the passage of the exhale, and you should hear it from the roof of your mouth.

3. Repeat several times.

Bhastrika: Bellows Breath

Bhastrika (*bah-STREE-kah*) is a powerful technique. Progress with it slowly to make the foundation strong. Bellows Breath brings heat to the body and is excellent for weight reduction, because it exercises the stomach and organs of the abdominal cavity. It clears energy, purifies the physical body, and opens up restrictions in the spine, permitting a freer energy flow. Put more emphasis on the exhale than on the inhale in this breath, just as a bellows "exhales" more forcefully than it "inhales."

A Yoga Minute

We inhale oxygen and exhale carbon dioxide. Trees and plants inhale carbon dioxide and exhale oxygen. Perfect harmony!

1. Exhale deeply and sharply, feeling your diaphragm muscle pull in your navel.

2. Inhale smoothly and exhale rapidly through your nose by continuing to force air out with sharp movements of your diaphragm. Don't worry about the inhale, which will take care of itself. Concentrate on the force of your exhalations.

3. Don't hold your breath between breaths. Aim for deep, quick movements of the diaphragm muscle. Remember, the inhalation will take little effort, especially as you practice this exercise and feel how the inhalation is a natural reflex following the exhalation.

4. Do 20 cycles, then hold your breath for a few seconds.

5. Repeat as many times as possible. If the strength of your exhalation begins to weaken, reduce the number of breaths in a cycle.

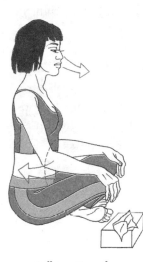

Bellows Breath.

Kapalabhati: Skull Shining

Kapalabhati (*KAH-pah-lah-BAH-tee*), or Skull Shining, is similar to Bellows Breath, except the inhale and exhale are evenly balanced with equal emphasis. This exercise has similar benefits but is like a calmer, easier, slower version. It is, therefore, more calming than bellows breath, which is more energizing. Because the skull consists of sinus passages, the technique is called Skull Shining, as it shines or clears the sinuses.

1. Feel your diaphragm muscle pull in your navel as you exhale deeply and sharply through your nose. Then pause, holding your breath, after the exhalation for just a second or two.

2. Inhale deeply through your nose, then exhale again through your nose with equal force, pushing the air out as you did before. Again, pause after the exhalation for a few seconds.

3. Pause between cycles. Do as many cycles as you can, spending one minute on each. Gradually increase the time of your meditation after the cycle.

Shitali: Cooling Breath

Shitali (*shee-TAH-lee*) is great for summer! This technique is healing to the body and cools it from excessive heat. It clears the eyes and ears, satisfies hunger and thirst, activates the liver, and improves digestion. Shitali involves rolling the tongue, then inhaling through it like a straw. Tongue rolling appears easy for some people and virtually impossible for others.

1. Roll your tongue into a tube and keep the tip of it slightly outside your mouth. (If you can't roll your tongue, just try to visualize the sides raising as well as you can.)

2. Draw in breath through your curled tongue as if you're sipping through a straw. Fill your lungs.

3. When your lungs are full, bring your tongue into your mouth and close your mouth. Hold your breath for a comfortable amount of time. As you do so, relax your tongue, mouth, and face.

4. Lower your chin slightly and retain the breath for a few seconds.

5. Exhale slowly through your nose.

6. Repeat several times.

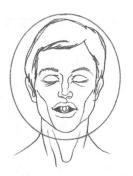

Breathing through your rolled tongue cools your body.

Nadi Shodhana: Alternate Nostril Breathing

Nadi shodhana (*NAH-dee shoh-DAH-nah*) balances the male/female or ha/tha within. It can be used to bring your emotions and your body back in balance. Gradually, the amount of time when both nostrils are closed should increase comfortably. Keep your finger movement to a minimum.

1. Sit in a meditative posture or comfortably in a chair or cross-legged on the floor. Close your eyes.

2. Cover your right nostril with your right thumb. Inhale through your left nostril.

3. Close your left nostril with the ring finger of your right hand. Your two middle fingers should be turned in toward your palm.

4. Hold both nostrils closed for as long as you can comfortably. Then release the right nostril and exhale through it.

5. Inhale through your right nostril, then close it again.

6. Hold both nostrils closed for as long as you can comfortably. Then exhale through your left nostril.

7. Inhale through your left nostril, close, exhale through your right nostril, and so on.

8. Repeat several times.

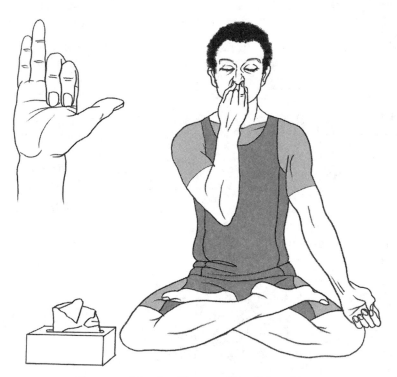

Finger position for Alternate Nostril Breathing.

Pranayama Plus

Many pranayama breathing exercises are performed while in a meditative seated pose, but others combine with yoga movements, are performed lying down, or otherwise enhance the prana flow by combining the movement of breath with the different movements and body positions.

Every movement and change of position you make affects the way prana moves through you. We think you'll enjoy these alternative pranayama exercises as much as we do!

Modified Mountain Breath

This pose is simple, but it helps you become more keenly aware of the way your breath feels in your body and how that feeling changes with simple changes in movement.

1. Stand in Mountain pose. Breathe normally, but focus your awareness on the way your breath feels as it expands your rib cage from all sides and the way it feels as it flows out of your body and your diaphragm collapses.

2. After a few minutes in Mountain, inhale and raise your arms above your head into a simple arms-raised version of Mountain pose.

3. Continue to breathe, but focus again on your rib cage and diaphragm, noticing how the breath feels different than it did before. How does the space in your chest change? How does the energy change? How does the flow of air change with each inhalation and exhalation? Notice how simply raising your arms can dramatically change your breath.

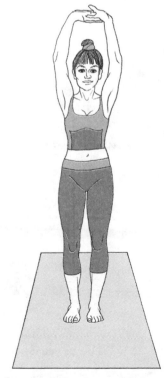

Feel how breathing changes simply by raising your arms in **Modified Mountain Breath.**

Namaste Breath

This exercise is a great way to energize in the morning and center yourself to prepare for the day ahead.

1. Sit in Lotus or Easy pose and relax for a moment.

2. Bring your hands together in front of your chest in prayer position (namaste).

3. Inhale strongly and lift your arms straight up over your head.

4. Exhale forcefully and bring your arms back down in front of your chest.

5. Continue to inhale while lifting your arms and exhale while lowering your arms, keeping your palms pressed together.

6. Repeat 12 times, pause, and sit for a moment, noticing how you feel.

7. Repeat 12 more times, pause, notice how you feel, then repeat for a third set of 12.

8. Have a great day!

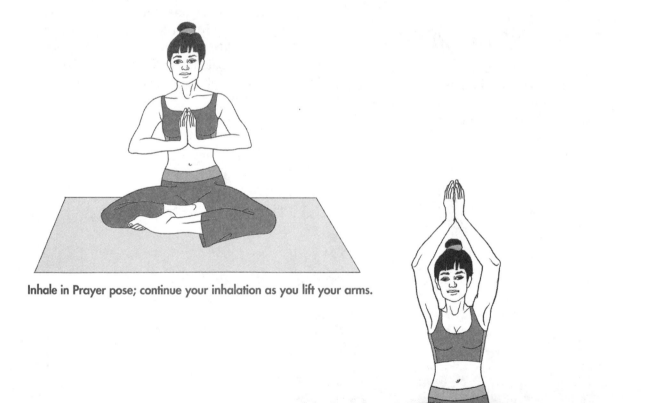

Inhale in Prayer pose; continue your inhalation as you lift your arms.

Exhale as you lower your lifted arms back down into Prayer pose.

Sun Breath

This exercise emphasizes the breath in an expanded or rising position and then in a contracted or seated position. As your body rises and sets like the sun, your breath expands and then contracts, letting prana move in and out of your body. Think day and night, light and dark, warm and cool, yang and yin. It's no coincidence that this exercise borrows the first two positions from yoga's popular Sun Salutation. When you practice Sun Salutation, remember to use the breath the way you use it in this exercise.

1. Stand with your feet together in Mountain pose.

2. Inhale and raise your arms above your head, expanding your rib cage in all directions and reaching as high as you can for a full, opening stretch.

3. Exhale as you bend over and reach toward the floor, slowly closing your rib cage like an accordion and pushing the air from your body with your diaphragm. Feel your front torso contracting and bend forward as far as you can.

4. Repeat several times slowly, then return to Mountain pose and notice how you feel.

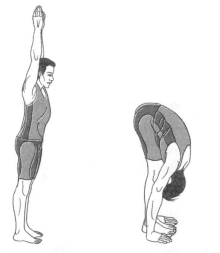

Sun Breath helps you feel the way your breath moves with a pose that expands on the inhale (left), then contracts on the exhale (right).

Weighted Breath

This exercise is like weightlifting for your diaphragm! You'll lie in Corpse pose but use a soft weight that will be comfortable on your stomach, such as a sandbag or a plastic-covered disc weight wrapped in a pillowcase or blanket, to help emphasize and add resistance to the diaphragm movement of the breath.

1. Lie in Corpse pose on your back on the floor, feet apart, and palms facing upward.

2. Place a weight on your stomach just under your ribs. Begin with a light weight of two to five pounds and work up to a ten-pound weight.

3. Concentrate on relaxing your entire body, but as you inhale, focus on lifting the weight with your diaphragm. As you exhale, notice how the weight helps press the breath out of your lungs.

4. Continue for several moments, then remove the weight and breathe normally in this relaxation pose. Feel the difference.

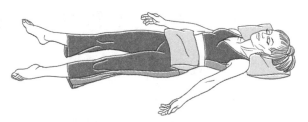

Weighted Breath strengthens your diaphragm muscle. You can also bend your knees, if that is more comfortable.

Yoga Ball Breath

Lying on a yoga ball instead of the floor opens the chest and the emotional center. Conscious breathing in this position helps suffuse the heart and the emotional center with prana, energizing and freeing your compassion and empathy. This pose also helps strengthen the small, stabilizing muscles of the torso as you balance on the ball.

1. Squat down and lean your back onto a yoga ball.

2. Feet on the ground, relax your legs, rolling the ball back until it sits in the middle of your back and you find a comfortable, stable balance for your body.

3. Center your spine on the ball. Separate your feet and plant them firmly on the floor for stability and balance.

4. Bring your attention to your breath. Feel how your diaphragm moves and how your rib cage expands and contracts while you rest on the yoga ball.

5. Breathe steadily; focus on the opening of your chest and imagine love and compassion flowing from your heart.

6. Stay here for several minutes; enjoy! Then slowly roll to be seated on the floor and lie back on the floor in Corpse pose. Feel how your body adjusts to accommodate the shape of the floor after lying on the yoga ball.

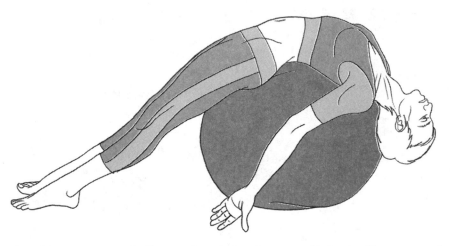

Breathing over a yoga ball opens the emotional center, suffusing it with energy and releasing compassion.

Crocodile Breath

As you lie on the floor in Crocodile pose, focus on how your torso expands outward from your back and let your whole body breathe! This exercise also uses the resistance of the floor to strengthen your diaphragm, as the front of your body moves outward with the inhalation against the floor.

1. Inhale slowly and deeply. Feel your rib cage expanding out of your back as you inhale. Exhale completely and feel your back sink back down.

2. Inhale again, but this time, focus on the front of your body and feel the resistance of the floor as your body expands with the inhalation. Let the resistance of the floor help press the breath out of your body with the exhalation.

3. Repeat, focusing alternately on the back and the front, for about 20 breaths.

4. Roll over onto your back into Corpse pose and breathe normally, feeling the difference in your breath.

We're confident you're feeling more energized by now. What a great way to prime your body for yoga postures—and life!

The Least You Need to Know

◆ Prana is the universal life force.

◆ Prana flows into the body via the breath.

◆ Pranayama are breathing techniques that, when practiced, result in better control of the mind and body.

◆ Let pranayama inspire you as it energizes your life.

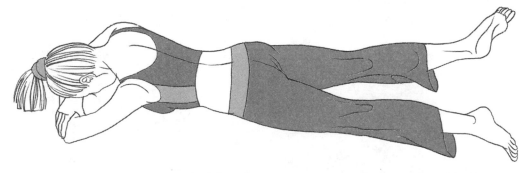

Crocodile Breath encourages "back breathing," because it uses the resistance of the floor to strengthen the diaphragm.

In This Chapter

- ◆ Why bend forward?

- ◆ Forward bends: Child, Standing Head to Knees, Feet Apart Side Angle, Sitting One Leg, Bound Half Lotus, Yoga Mudra, Boat, Tortoise

- ◆ An all-around stretch: Downward Facing Dog

- ◆ Modifications, challenges, and other tips to improve your yoga practice

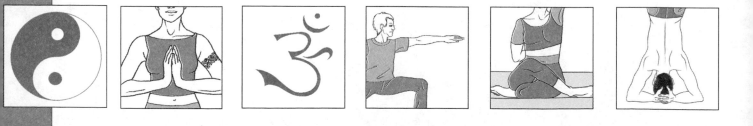

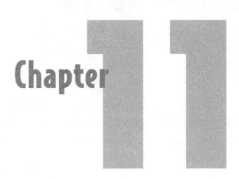

Chapter **11**

Take the Forward Path

Forward bends are among some of the most revitalizing poses, from the comfort of Child's pose to the refreshing stretch of Downward Facing Dog, and we're not just saying that because we like kids and dogs. Many of these poses activate your Venus chakra, replenishing your heart center. They can also relieve lower back pain.

Forward bends also help us focus inward, quieting our busy minds. As your body bends forward, it folds your heart into its center and your emotional mind begins to quiet down. We all need a little peace and quiet sometimes, and forward bends help us to move in this direction.

Forward-Bending Basics

In forward bends, always bend from the hips, not the waist. Bend forward slightly and place your hands on your hip joints at the top of your thighs to feel the movement there.

Forward bends are great for stretching out and loosening the lower back muscles and also for lengthening the hamstrings. Believe it or not, the leg muscles, especially the *gluteus maximus* (the muscles of the derrière) often hold more stress than any other muscle group in the body! Forward bends help you reach that inner place where you can allow your lower back and hamstrings to relax and become fluid.

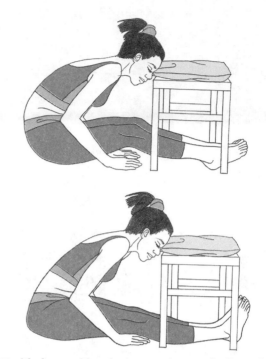

Modify forward bends using a chair and pillows for support. Bend from the hips and feel the slow, consistent release in the hip joints. Bend knees if the back is tight, and slowly the spine will lengthen.

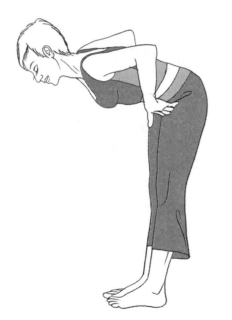

When bending forward, place your fingertips at the hip joints, where your thighs and hips meet. Bend forward and gently press in to more closely feel the movement forward from this point.

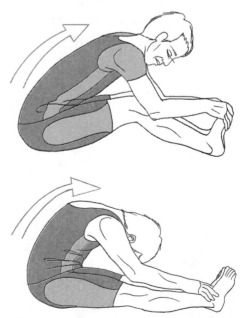

If your hamstrings are tight, let your knees bend and focus on lengthening your spine over your legs. Avoid the hunched, curved back that comes from trying to keep the legs straight. Try moving forward from the hips instead of the waist for a longer stretch.

Mudhasana: Child's Pose

Child's pose makes you feel safe and nurtured, as if you were still in the womb. Mudhasana (*moo-DAH-sah-nah*) activates your fourth and fifth chakras (located behind your heart and at the base of your skull, respectively), relieves lower back pain, and improves your complexion. It also stimulates respiration because it compresses your diaphragm.

1. Sit back on your heels, then bring your forehead to the floor.

2. Rest your arms alongside your body with your palms facing upward. The pose should feel completely relaxing.

3. Breathe deeply. Feel your diaphragm rising and sinking with each breath, like a baby's tummy.

Easing into the Pose

When practicing Child's pose, if you are not resting back on your heels, you can place pillows or a blanket under your head to help lengthen your back. If you are not touching your heels, cross your arms beneath your head. Also, if you feel strain in your knees, you may place a pillow or blanket in the crease of the back of the knees, between your thighs and calves.

Continuing the Challenge: Elongated Child's Pose

To modify this pose, stretch your arms out in front of you. Feel your spine lengthen as you relax into this elongated version of Child's pose. If you curl your toes under, it will help you move easily into Downward Facing Dog.

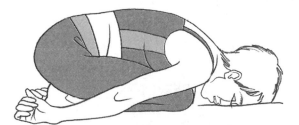

Child's pose.

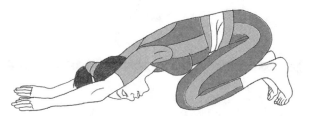

Child's pose variation with outstretched arms.

Forward Bend with V-Legs Pose

We love this forward bend because it feels so good! It gives a deep stretch to the hamstrings and muscles of the inner thighs.

1. Spread your feet about four to five feet apart, toes pointed forward or slightly inward.

2. Exhale and bend slowly forward, dropping your head between your legs as you run your hands down each leg for support.

3. Go as far as you can to feel the stretch, but not so far as to cause pain.

Easing into the Pose

As you bend down in this pose, grasp your thighs, calves, or ankles with your hands. Or rest your hands or forearms on the ground under your head. Clasp your elbows with your hands to stabilize your upper body on the ground if you can reach that far. If you have very flexible hamstrings, you might even be able to rest your head on your forearms or the floor. Once this pose is comfortable, it is very relaxing and stabilizing because you are forming a tripod with your two feet and your joined forearms and head.

Continuing the Challenge

You can check your quadriceps tone in this pose. While holding Forward Bend with V-Legs, tense your thigh (quadriceps) muscles, lifting your kneecaps with the contraction. See how long you can hold this tension in your thigh muscles. If you can only hold it for a few seconds, you need to build strength in your quads. Warrior poses are good for this. On the other hand, if your quadriceps muscles are rock-hard and you can't seem to move your knee caps, try poses that stretch the quads, such as Hero or Bridge pose.

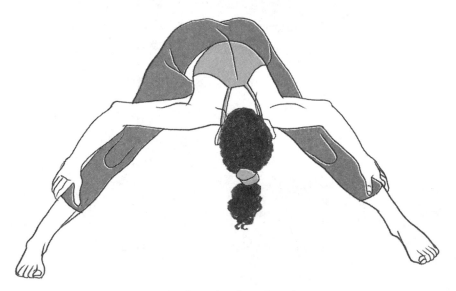

Forward Bend with V-Legs pose.

Uttanasana: Standing Head to Knees Pose

Uttanasana (*OOH-tah-NAH-sah-nah*) stretches the entire back of your body. It also tones your abdomen, decreases bloating, refreshes your mind, and clears your head. Forward bends are also conducive to relaxation and sleep, so a few forward bends followed by Corpse pose in the evenings are a great way to wind down before sleep.

1. Stand with your feet together. Inhale and raise your arms overhead.

2. Exhale and bend forward at your hips. (Remember not to bend at the waist, curving your back!) Try to bend at your hip joints to keep your heart open as you move forward. Think of touching your heart to your knees. Keep your knees slightly bent and slowly straighten them as your back comfort permits.

3. Be careful not to rock your weight back to your heels. Keep your weight evenly distributed over your feet. Keep lengthening without turning your feet out. Move forward from your hips instead of your waist, lengthening through your lower back. Don't force your head toward your knees—let gravity do the work as your head and neck stay relaxed. Don't be concerned with how far you bend. Focus on how open your heart can become as you "lift" forward.

Easing into the Pose: Bending Your Knees

In forward bends, you might have to bend your knees, and that's fine! Your body's flexibility doesn't determine the benefits of this pose; the bend from the hips does the trick. As you become more flexible, you'll be able to grasp your big toes with your index fingers. For those who can fold in half, give yourselves a hug!

Easing into the Pose: Support

If Standing Head to Knees is too intense for you, try relaxing into this pose using books, and/or foam or wooden blocks as props. Yoga blocks are available in many stores that sell fitness equipment. Wise yogis that we are, we use books! Rest each hand on a book, and rest your head on a stack of books reaching to a comfortable height for your flexibility.

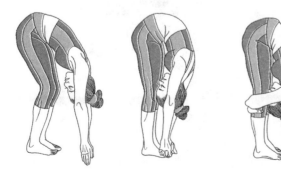

Standing Head to Knees pose.

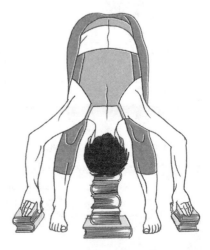

Use support books to help with balance and stability, if you need them.

Parshvottanasana: Feet Apart Side Angle Pose

In parshvottanasana (*PARSH-voh-tah-NAH-sah-nah*), you will tone your abdomen; straighten drooping shoulders; and make your hips, spine, and wrists more flexible.

1. Stand with your feet three to four feet apart. Turn one foot out so it is perpendicular with the other foot, the heel of your turned foot lining up with the arch of your straight foot. Turn your body to face your turned-out foot.

2. Bring your hands into the namaste or prayer position behind your back with your fingers pointing up. If this is too difficult, simply clasp your hands behind your back or keep your hands at your sides as you move forward.

3. Inhale, lengthen your spine upward, then exhale, bringing your heart toward your front knee.

4. Imagine your chest, rather than your head, moving toward your knees to help lengthen your spine and prevent rounding your back. Keep breathing throughout this pose.

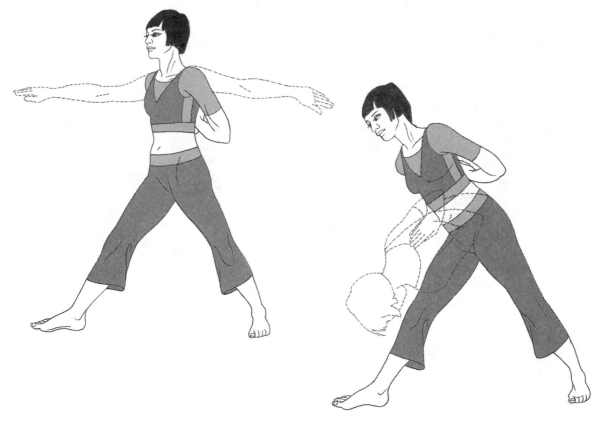

Feet Apart Side Angle pose.

Janu Shirshasana: Sitting One Leg Pose

In janu shirshasana (*JAH-noo shur-SHAH-sah-nah*), *janu* means "knee," and *shirsha* means "head." You might guess that this pose, then, involves bringing the head and knees together. You're right! Sitting One Leg pose tones your abdomen, liver, spleen, and kidneys. It quiets your mind and aids digestion, as well as stretching and strengthening your lower back and chest. Men suffering from an enlarged prostate will benefit from this pose as well.

Remember, it's okay to bend your knees! As you become more flexible, you'll be able to straighten your leg and grasp your foot with your hands.

1. Sit on the floor with your left leg straight in front of you, toes pointed upward. Your right leg should be bent in toward the straight leg.

2. Raise your hands over your head, exhale, and slowly bend forward over your straight leg. Lengthen your spine and open your heart as you move forward.

3. Hold the stretch, then inhale as you rise back up. Repeat on the other side.

> **Wise Yogi Tells Us**
>
> If you feel stress on your back doing the Sitting One Leg pose, bend the knee you are reaching toward. Angle your body directly over this knee. Release any competitive thoughts. Forget your goals and open your heart. Bend at your hips, not your waist. Don't hurry, be patient with yourself. Slowly your legs and hips will open.

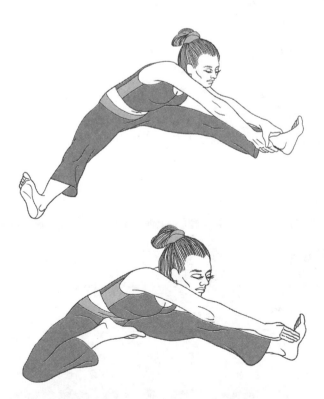

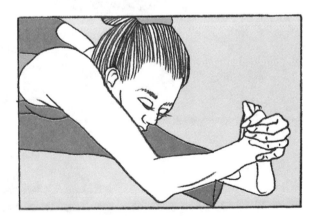

Sitting One Leg pose.

Paschimothanasana: Sitting Forward Bend Pose

Sitting Forward Bend helps the spine be more flexible as it stretches the entire back of your body from your neck to your calf.

1. Sit with your legs stretched out in front of you, feet together and relaxed.

2. Inhale and bend forward, folding your torso over your thighs and reaching your hands toward your feet. Don't strain your head toward your knees. Instead, keep your head up and gently ease your chest toward your thighs. When you have pulled yourself down as far as you can, relax your head down.

3. If you can reach your feet, flex them and hook your index fingers around your big toes. Gently pull to increase the stretch. If you can't reach that far, just ease your hands down your legs as far as you can. Keep your head in line with your spine.

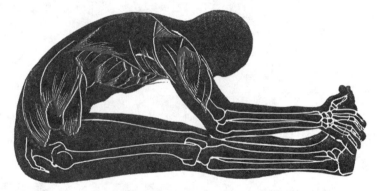

This is how your musculoskeletal system looks in Sitting Forward Bend.

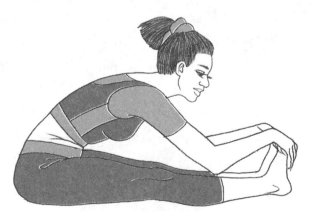

Sitting Forward Bend.

Ardha Baddha Padma Pashchimottanasana: Bound Half Lotus Pose

Ardha baddha padma pashchimottanasana (*AHR-dah BAH-dah PAHD-mah PAH-shih-moh-tah-NAH-sah-nah*) is identical to Sitting One Leg pose, except that the foot of your bent leg is in a Half Lotus position, with one foot placed on the opposite thigh.

If this pose seems impossible, be patient. The pose will come.

1. Sit on the floor with one leg in front of you (as in Sitting One Leg pose) and the other leg bent, foot placed on your opposite thigh in Half Lotus.

2. Bring your arm around your back and connect your hand to this foot.

3. Face your upper torso directly over your extended leg. Open your chest, exhale, and slowly bend forward. Repeat on the other side.

Ouch!

Not every pose is for every body. Be patient and kind with your body, and your body will respond accordingly. You will be amazed at the power of TLC (tender loving care)!

Easing into the Pose: Hamstring Stretch

Ease into Bound Half Lotus by sitting with one leg tucked into a Half Easy pose. Stretch your hamstring by looping a towel or strap around your foot and pulling gently rather than bending your body forward. Keep your back straight and your neck in line with your spine.

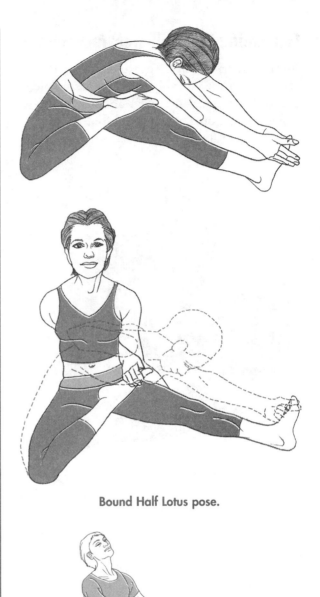

Bound Half Lotus pose.

Stretch your hamstrings using a strap and pulling gently as you keep your back straight and neck in line with your spine.

Continuing the Challenge: Archer Pose

For a hamstring and inner thigh stretch that also helps make your hip joints more mobile, try Archer pose, akarna dhanurasana. From Bound Half Lotus, pick up the foot of your folded leg with the hand on the same side of your body and lift it gently by the ball of the foot toward your ear. Keep your elbow lifted. With your other hand, reach straight out toward the toe of your straight leg, grasping it if you can. Your body becomes bow, arrow, archer—bodymindspirit. Enjoy the lovely stretch!

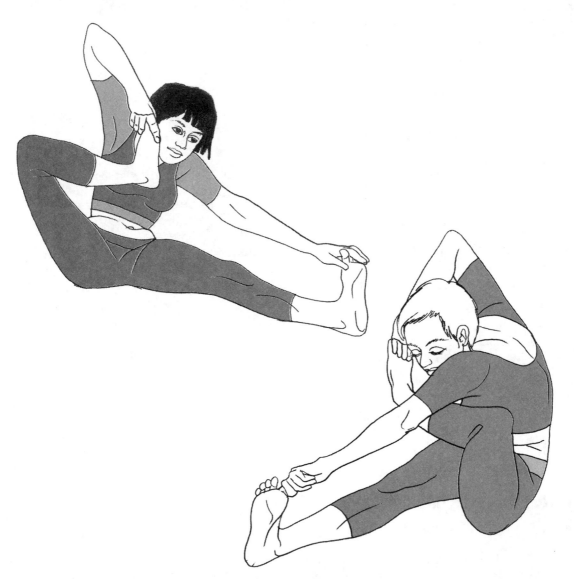

Adjust your feet from Bound Half Lotus into Archer pose for a great hamstring stretch that adds mobility to your hip joints.

Continuing the Challenge: Foot-to-Head Pose

From Archer, you can give your hips an even greater stretch with Foot-to-Head pose, eka pada sirasana, but don't push this until you are flexible enough. From Archer pose, bend your outstretched knee and tuck your foot close to your body as in Easy pose, but take the foot you have in your raised hand and gently ease it behind your head so your heel rests on the opposite shoulder, toes pointed upward. Now both hands are free to rest in Prayer pose (namaste). Breathe and hold for several moments, then gently raise your foot and place it back down into Full Easy pose.

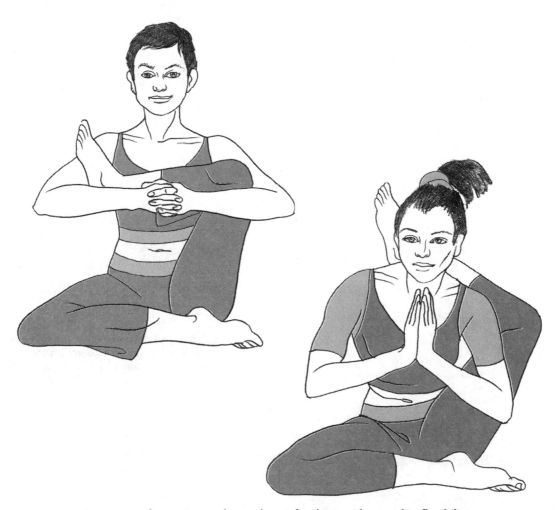

Foot-to-Head pose is an advanced pose for those with great hip flexibility.

Yoga Mudra: Ego Be Gone!

Yoga Mudra (*YOH-gah MOO-drah*) is a symbol of unity. This important pose inspires feelings of devotion and humility. It also stretches your legs and hips, opens your shoulders, and aids the gastrointestinal tract. To add a challenge to this pose, bring your hands into namaste behind your back.

1. Sit cross-legged or in Kneeling pose.

2. Move your arms behind your back, clasp your hands, and lower your head to the floor.

3. Keeping your arms straight, lift your clasped hands up over your head until your arms are perpendicular to the floor.

Wise Yogi Tells Us

Just a friendly reminder to your ego: Take a hike! When performing any yoga pose, especially more difficult poses, don't allow your ego to take over. If you find yourself thinking *Look at me touching the floor!* or *Wow, I'm so good at this!* re-adjust your thoughts. The aim of yoga is to release the ego, not to feed it. Feel how the posture you're holding helps your mind become clear and your heart more open.

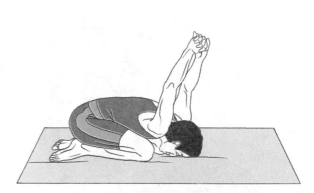

If you can't bring your hands into a namaste position behind your back, interlace your fingers and bring your arms up behind you. This opens the shoulder area so that eventually your hands will reach easily into namaste.

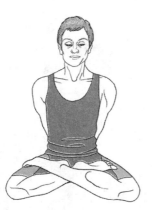

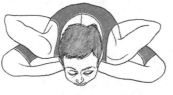

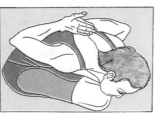

Yoga Mudra pose.

Naukasana: Boat Pose

A yogi holding naukasana (*now-KAH-sah-nah*) looks like a boat bobbing on the waves, and *nauka* literally means "ship." Boat pose tones your stomach and intestines, strengthens your back, and activates your third chakra (located behind your navel).

In Boat pose, don't hold your breath as you are balancing. Your feet may fall to the floor at first. Whether you are doing Full Boat pose or Half Boat pose, keep your leg position steady and your knees together.

1. For Full Boat pose, sit on the floor with your knees bent in front of you and your arms holding your knees.

2. Lean back to about a 45-degr bring your feet off the floor, and b on your tailbone.

3. Raise your feet straight up in the air so your body forms a V shape. For balance, extend your arms straight out, parallel to the floor at about knee level.

4. Imagine you are bobbing on top of the water like a little buoy.

If balancing in Full Boat pose is too difficult at first, start with Half Boat pose. Keep your knees bent, but instead of raising your feet all the way up, raise them to a right angle to the floor. Keep your knees together. Bring your hands alongside your feet with your palms facing in.

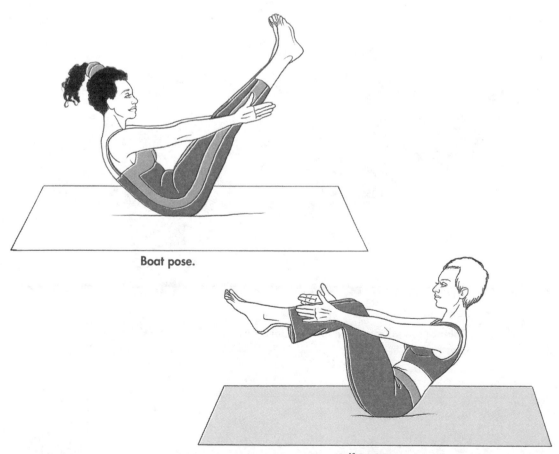

Boat pose.

Half Boat pose.

Santulangasana: Balancing Chalice Pose

This challenging balance pose is great for improving concentration and also strengthens the abdomen and hips.

1. Begin in Easy pose with your back straight and your head lifted.

2. Grasp one ankle with your hand and inhale as you straighten your leg to the side. Exhale as you slowly bring the leg in front of you.

3. Grasp the other ankle with your other hand and inhale as you straighten the second leg to the side, then exhale as you slowly bring it forward. Your legs should form a V, your arms are straight and strong, and your back stays straight with head lifted.

4. Focus on a single point in front of you to help you balance, and hold as long as your abdominal strength allows or for a few controlled breaths.

5. Release your legs back down into Easy pose and breathe, resting for a moment to feel the difference between balanced sitting and stable sitting.

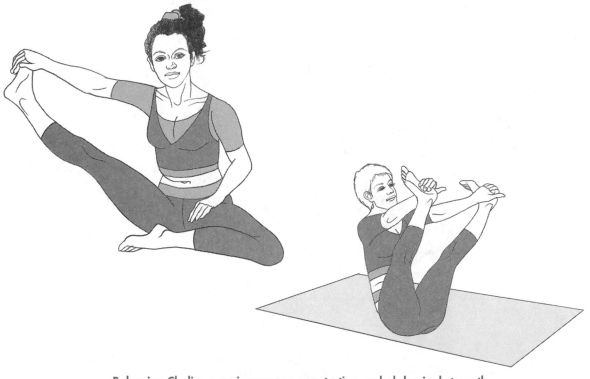

Balancing Chalice pose improves concentration and abdominal strength.

Kurmasana: Tortoise Pose

You'll look like a tortoise when you practice kurmasana (*koohr-MAH-sah-nah*). This pose keeps your lumbar limber! (In other words, it makes your lower spine more flexible.) It also strengthens your neck, massages your thyroid, aids digestion, and rejuvenates your nervous system. Take it slowly—just like a tortoise!

Does Tortoise pose seem impossible? Simply lower yourself as far as you can, let the corners of your mouth turn upward like a cute little turtle, and enjoy the journey to the floor, even if it takes many, many yoga practices to extend as big as a tortoise. Tortoises are not in a hurry. They live long lives!

1. Sit with your legs extended in front of you in a V shape. Bend your knees just slightly, and slide your arms under your knees with your palms on the floor.

2. Slowly straighten your legs again to hold your arms against the floor and bring your chest forward. Your chin will eventually reach the floor.

A Yoga Minute

Hypothyroidism, the underproduction of the thyroid hormone, is a common condition and might be the underlying cause of many recurring illnesses and chronic fatigue. Symptoms of an underactive thyroid include fatigue, weight gain, weakness, dry skin, hair loss, recurrent infections, depression, and intolerance to cold. So, for a nice thyroid massage, try Tortoise pose.

Tortoise pose.

Adho Mukha Shvanasana: Downward Facing Dog Pose

Another pose named after the esteemed canine. Downward Facing Dog, adho mukha shvana-sana (*AH-doh MOO-kah shvah-NAH-sah-nah*), brings heat to your body, strengthens and stretches your spine, and gives your heart a rest.

This is one of the better-known yoga poses—maybe because it feels so great to do it! Downward Facing Dog is easily adjustable for any flexibility level. You can reach down to the floor—or even to the seat of a firmly anchored chair—if you can't quite make it all the way down. Or if you are very flexible, you can press all the way down to the floor with your palms and your heels while pushing your hips up. *Ahh*, doesn't that feel great?

If you have trouble with this pose because of tight hamstrings, spend extra yoga time on Sitting Forward Bends to loosen the back of your legs. If Downward Facing Dog hurts your wrists, you might not be balancing your weight evenly. Try placing a rolled-up towel or blanket under the heel of each hand. This will take some of the pressure off your wrists. Then try to shift your weight back onto the heels of your feet. (All these heels! We definitely are talking about dogs!) Hold the pose only as long as you are comfortable. Little by little, your balance will shift, and this pose will eventually become quite soothing.

Ouch!

If your back is sore or tight, definitely keep your knees bent. Focus on spine lengthening, instead of legs straightening.

It might also help to concentrate on stretching out your lower back. Instead of rounding it, lengthen it. Remember the way your back is stretched out in Child's pose? Think about lifting your tailbone to the sky. If necessary, keep your knees slightly bent to return a natural curve to your lower back. When you are flexible and strong enough to perform Downward Facing Dog fully and peacefully, you will place as much weight on your feet as you do on your hands. To get this feeling of the full pose, have a partner lift your hips up and shift your weight back to center, as shown in the following illustration.

1. Get down on your hands and knees. Lift your tailbone up, bringing your knees off the floor so your body forms an upside-down V, with your palms and the balls of your feet touching the floor.

2. Bring your head down and your hips up. Keep your knees bent at first, then slowly bring your heels to the floor and straighten your legs. No rush to straighten those legs. With dedicated practice, they will open in their own time. Breathe and hold for as long as it feels good.

3. Have a partner check your hips to make sure they are straight rather than listing to one side and weight is evenly distributed between your legs and arms.

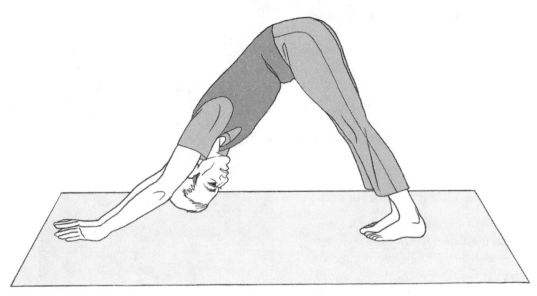

Downward Facing Dog pose.

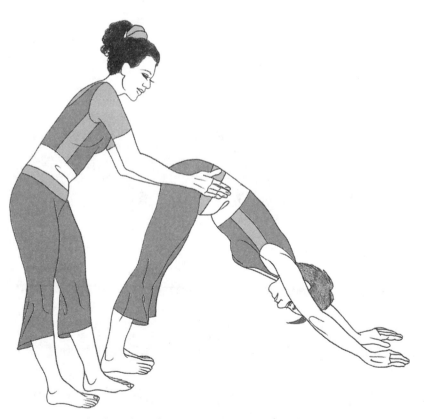

Checking hip alignment in Downward Facing Dog.

Continuing the Challenge: Heel Toe Stretches

For an extra foot and calf stretch in Downward Facing Dog, alternately bend one leg and push into the other leg, feeling your heel powering into the ground and pushing up with your hips for a deep, one-leg isolation stretch. Repeat on the other side.

Continuing the Challenge: Heel Lift

To strengthen your leg muscles and improve your balance, try a heel lift in Downward Facing Dog. Exhale and bend your knees slightly and lift your heels off the ground. Feel your spine lengthen. Hold for a few seconds, then inhale and lower your heels back to the ground, keeping the spine elongated. Repeat several times.

Continuing the Challenge: Elbow Dog

To make Downward Facing Dog even more challenging, combine it with Elbow Dog, which deepens the leg stretch as it strengthens your shoulders and upper arms. From Downward Facing Dog pose, slowly lower yourself down onto your forearms, bringing your elbows to the ground. The more you do this pose, the more flexibility you will gain in your calves and hamstrings.

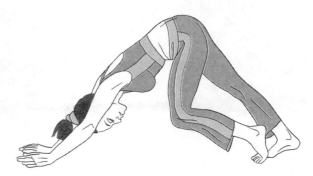

Heel/toe alternate stretches in Downward Facing Dog.

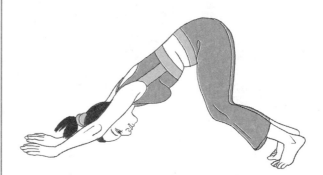

Heel Lift in Downward Facing Dog.

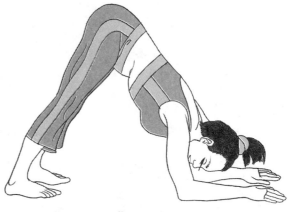

Elbow Dog.

Feeling worn out yet? The next chapter will give you a chance to let your body really relax so all that work can take effect. Corpse pose is, paradoxically, the easiest and the most challenging yoga pose of all. Read on to learn more, and prepare to get really, really relaxed.

The Least You Need to Know

◆ Forward-bending postures—such as Standing Head to Knees, Feet Apart Side Angle, Sitting One Leg, Bound Half Lotus, Yoga Mudra, Boat, Half Boat, Tortoise, and Downward Facing Dog—help you internalize and quiet your mind.

◆ Many forward bends are good for replenishing, revitalizing, and reawakening your heart center.

◆ Forward bends are great for loosening your lower back and stretching out your hamstrings.

◆ Forward bends and backbends balance each other and should be practiced together.

In This Chapter

◆ Why a pose named after a corpse is the most important of all the poses

◆ More on Om

◆ How to relax and stop thinking

◆ Finding peace at last!

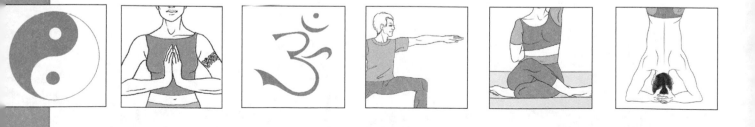

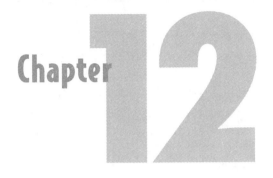

Chapter 12

Dead to the World

Of all the yoga poses, shavasana (*shah-VAH-sah-nah*), also known as Corpse pose, is the most important. *Shava* means "corpse," and just as it sounds, Corpse pose consists of lying on the floor in complete relaxation, still, peaceful, and corpselike. "How can lying on the floor be important?" you might ask. Or better yet, "How can imitating a corpse be important?"

Both good questions! Here's a good answer: the essence of peace comes from within, not from without. Shavasana's goal is to relax the body so completely that the body becomes irrelevant, as if it were deceased. With the body "gone," the mind is set free to blossom. Shavasana sinks into that space between life and the beyond.

It's a yoga paradox that a pose that suggests death is the way to learn to live. But the Corpse pose brings your focus inward, beyond all the ego trappings of who you think you are and to the real you. Mastering shavasana is mastering knowledge of the real you.

Relaxing the Bodymind in Corpse Pose

So you see, there's more to this pose than lying on the floor. It's all about focus. So let's practice!

For some people, lying on a firm floor and/or lying flat on their backs is uncomfortable, even painful. If this sounds like you, try Supported Corpse pose. Lie on the floor with a blanket or small pillow under your head and neck. Keep your arms at your sides, palms up, but rest your knees, lower legs, and feet on a chair so your legs are bent at a right angle. Rest, breathe, and relax.

1. Lie comfortably on your back on the floor, and separate your legs so your feet are two to three feet apart. Let your toes fall out to the sides. Close your eyes.

2. Separate your arms so each hand is two to three feet from your body, with each palm facing upward.

3. Roll your head from side to side, releasing tension in your neck.

4. Roll your shoulders down and away from your ears.

5. Allow your attention to travel up and down your body, scanning for tight spots or contracted muscles. When you find a tight spot, gently tell the area to relax (out loud, if it helps). Place a pillow under your knees or head if this helps you relax.

6. Repeat your body scan until your body is relaxed in every area.

7. Now bring your attention to your breath. Listen to your breath. Don't try to control it. Simply observe it. Feel it flowing in and out of you. Make the sound and feel of your breath the sole focus of your attention.

8. If part of your body starts to tense up, redirect your mind to the tense area and focus on relaxing it again. Then return to the breath.

9. As thoughts pop into your mind, let them pass back out of your mind. Imagine they are soap bubbles. Allow your breath to blow them away softly, up into the sky.

10. Come back to the breath. Back to the breath. To the breath. The breath. Breath. Om.

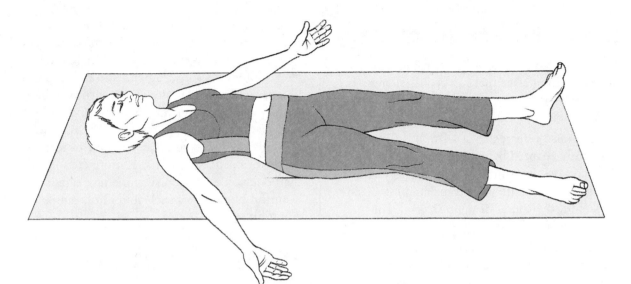

Shavasana: Yoga's Corpse pose.

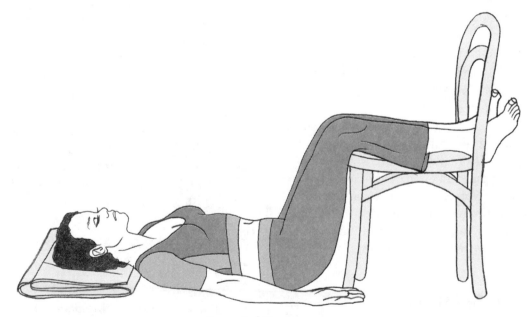

Supported Corpse pose.

One for All, and All for Om!

Maybe lying on the floor is no problem for you, but everything after that is a real challenge. It isn't easy to relax, let alone clear the mind. Om to the rescue!

Aum (also referred to as "Om") is the sound frequently chanted by yogis, because it is an all-encompassing sound. According to yogic thought, if all of life were translated into a single sound, the sound of the universe, that sound would be *Aum*.

Try saying the sound now, right where you are. Take a deep breath, breathing from your diaphragm, and sing out the *o* sound as long as you can without your voice faltering. Don't be afraid to put some sound and strength behind it. If you're worried about keeping your volume down too much, you might not give the sound the breath support it requires. Stay strong and sing out the sound, then slowly let the vowel sounds come to a close in a resonating, vibrating *mmmmm* sound.

Now take a breath, close your eyes, and try it again. Let the sound stretch out for as long as you can with the support of a deep breath. Use up all your breath, but don't strain yourself. Doesn't that feel good? Do it again if you'd like to. Notice how, when your entire body is vibrating with that sound, it's easier to concentrate on your breath and the sound. Notice that the distracting thoughts go away.

A Yoga Minute

According to an eyewitness account, Gandhi's last words to his assailant as he fell to the ground on January 30, 1948 from a gunshot wound were "Rama, Rama," which means "Praise God." This is the essence of yoga: to have one's thoughts continuously uplifted, even (especially!) in the transition from one existence to another.

Also notice how much saying *Aum* sounds like "amen," the word used at the end of prayers or hymns. Have you ever noticed that when a chorus of voices sings "amen," the voices often bloom from a single note into a harmony, like a multi-petalled flower opening in sound? Think how nicely this concept fits into the yogic way of thinking. Many voices harmonize to form a single, beautiful sound that is more complete than one voice alone, just as the universe is a beautiful blending of each soul into a single vibration.

When the Easiest Is the Hardest

Some of you might still be stuck on the idea that shavasana is the most important of all the postures. "How hard can it be?" you might wonder. How hard can it be to lie on the floor and relax? Actually, shavasana is the most challenging pose, even though it seems, at first, to be the easiest.

The true challenge with shavasana is not physical but mental—a state of total relaxation. It's possible to lie in a perfect shavasana without coming close to a yogic state of mind. The ideal state of shavasana is that the body is merely a shell, while the soul is in a state of perfect union with the Universe.

Beneath the Layers: The Body

Shavasana is about opening up and letting go, but it's a process. First you release tension in your body, then you release the tensions of the mind. Within the body, you relax little by little. The following exercises focus on releasing and relaxing your lower body, upper body, and face.

The Lower Body

It's good to ease into shavasana by focusing relaxation on the lower body first. Here's how:

1. Tighten one foot, curling your toes and contracting your foot muscles for a few seconds. Release and feel the tension flowing from your foot.

2. Flex your ankle and tighten your calf, then relax both.

3. Lift your entire leg two inches off the ground. Tense your leg, especially your large thigh muscle. Squeeze! Then let your leg fall to the ground. With the release, imagine all the tension falling away.

4. Repeat these steps with your other foot and leg.

5. Lift your hips two inches off the floor and squeeze your buttocks as tightly as you can for several seconds. Then release the contraction and drop your hips back down. Feel all the tight areas releasing and relaxing. Your hip joints should feel loose and your buttocks muscles completely relaxed.

Ouch!

If lying flat on the floor is uncomfortable for your back, put pillows or blankets under your knees. This protects your lower back from undue strain. If your head or neck is uncomfortable, rest your head or neck on a small pillow, but make sure your throat feels open. Too many pillows could block the flow of energy through your neck; too few pillows could cause your neck to overstrain backward. If you have low blood pressure and your feet get cold, wear socks. Strive for a feeling of openness in all parts of your body.

The Upper Body

Now, let's focus on the upper body:

1. Contract your stomach muscles as tightly as you can, then release them.

2. Lift one arm about two inches off the floor. Squeeze your hand into a fist and hold it tightly. Flex your arm muscles for several seconds, then relax your entire arm and let it fall. Feel stress and tightness flowing down your arm and out the ends of your fingers. Repeat with your other arm.

3. Tighten your chest muscles, then release them. As you release them, try to feel your heartbeat. Gently tell your heart to relax, slow down, and rest.

4. Bring your shoulders up to your ears, tensing your shoulders for several seconds. Release them and feel all the stress dropping away. Many people carry tension in their shoulders. You might want to do this several times until your shoulders feel truly loose.

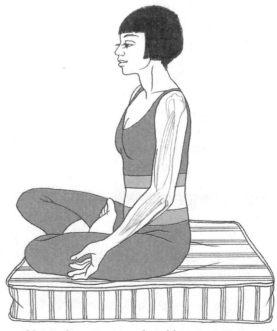

If lying down is uncomfortable, try sitting upright and tensing then relaxing muscles to begin a seated shavasana journey.

The Ultimate Facial

And now for the rest of you:

1. Lift your head two inches off the ground. Tense all your neck and facial muscles, scrunching up your face like a prune. Purse your lips and imagine you are trying to bring every part of your face to your nose. Release and lower your head.

2. Raise your head again, and open your eyes and mouth as wide as you possibly can. Stick your tongue out as far as you can. Really stretch your face for several seconds, then relax and lower your head to the ground.

3. Roll your head slowly and gently from one side to the other.

4. One at a time, scan your senses. First, notice what you can taste. Now let it go. Take your mind away from your taste buds. Next, notice what you can smell, then release your sense of smell. Notice everything your body is touching, then imagine you are floating and can't feel anything. Let go of your sense of sight (your eyes should already be closed) by releasing all tension around your eyes. Lastly, what can you hear? Observe, then let this go, too.

5. Now go back over each body part again, but this time, instead of physically tensing and releasing your muscles, mentally instruct each part to relax. Really focus on each area, one at a time, and coax it to release all pain and tension.

6. Now you should feel very, very relaxed and internalized. Mentally scan your body a few more times, seeking out pockets of stress and releasing them with the exhale.

Beneath the Layers: The Mind

The mind can be just as distracting as the body when it comes to true relaxation—maybe more so! So what's an active-minded person to do? Simple: stop thinking.

But this idea requires just as much effort—or maybe more—than the most complicated yoga posture. After all, we *are* our minds—aren't we? Not according to yogic philosophy. Wise yogis tell us that we aren't our bodies or our minds at all. These are merely tools to help free our souls and bring them into fuller and more unifying consciousness.

As you rest in shavasana, think of your mind as merely a tool that helps you with many tasks. During shavasana, it's time to put the tools away. Put away your thoughts. Let them go. You can always pick them up again later.

Dream a Little Dream

Imagine waking up one morning with the memory of a beautiful dream. In the dream, you are walking through your home, and everything is familiar until you come upon a door you've never noticed before. You open the door and step through it into a new universe. Pure beauty surrounds you, and you are filled with a sense of bliss. You realize that you are perfect. You have no faults, no sins, no shortcomings, no guilt. You are a being of pure light, and the whimsically lovely universe that encompasses you is also you. Love radiates from you and into you. You vaguely remember the comparatively ponderous and painful life of striving on the other side of the door through which you came, but as you look behind you, the door is gone, and you realize that other life was just a dream.

And then you wake up. Which was real and which was the dream? Yogic philosophy says that this life we lead in these earthbound bodies and minds is the dream, and that pure bliss is the reality. Yoga helps us wake from this dream.

Still, this dream exists for a reason, and we all move through this dream called life to learn about our souls.

Maybe the word *dream* throws you off, and maybe the word *illusion* is more accurate. Yogic thought says that anything that isn't eternal and blissful is an illusion. Shavasana helps us work past our bodies and dig through our thoughts until we unearth the jewel that is cosmic consciousness.

Give Your Mind a Breather

But to get practical, think of shavasana as giving your mind a breather, the same way you would give yourself a vacation or you would hire a babysitter for a night out. Giving yourself a break is rejuvenating and gives you a new perspective on life. That's what shavasana does for your mind—and you can do it every day.

> **Wise Yogi Tells Us**
>
> "Do not take life's experiences too seriously. Above all, do not let them hurt you, for in reality, they are nothing but dream experiences. ... If circumstances are bad and you have to bear them, do not make them a part of yourself. Play your part in life, but never forget that it is only a role."
>
> —Paramahansa Yogananda

Soaring Beyond

Let shavasana become a part of your workout, and take it just as seriously as any other posture— even *more* seriously. Your body will learn how to release all its tensions and will benefit even more from the other postures because of its time spent in shavasana. Your spirit, too, will learn how to soar beyond the limits of its "container." Now *that's* a powerful skill!

The Least You Need to Know

- If you practice only one yoga pose, practice shavasana.
- Mastering shavasana can require more discipline than the most physically demanding yoga postures!
- In shavasana, first you consciously relax your body, then you consciously relax your mind.
- Learning to quiet your mind and remove scattered thinking will bring you peace.

In This Part

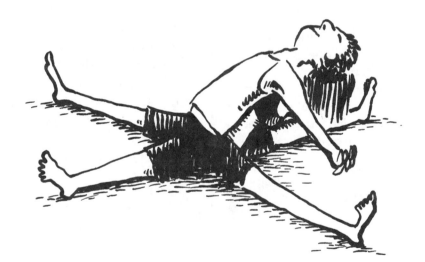

Part 4

Living Yoga

Yoga is a way of life. You'll find it's an essential building block for your relationships and your overall health. In this part, you'll find out how to do yoga with a partner and how to do it with your children. And if you are a woman, we have some advice to help you meet unique female challenges, from premenstrual syndrome to postpartum depression to menopause. Finally, we'll look at the many ways yoga can be used for healing.

In This Chapter

- ◆ How yoga is different when practiced in pairs
- ◆ Great postures for partners
- ◆ How doing yoga poses together can deepen relationships
- ◆ Why yoga is great for the whole family

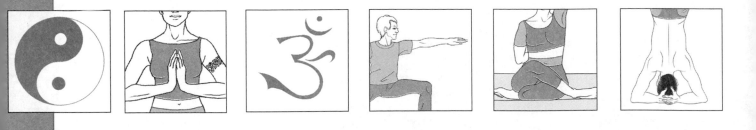

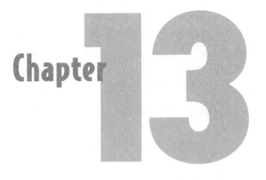

Chapter 13

Yoga for Two—or More!

Yoga is primarily a solitary and self-reflective pursuit, but it can be very rewarding to practice it with someone else. Why? Because practicing with someone special can encourage us to continue on. Even though yoga is ultimately a solitary pursuit, the journey can certainly involve enthusiastic sharing. Especially when we begin the study of yoga, poses you perform alone can be more intensely experienced when someone else helps you. When you take the journey hand in hand, practicing yoga with a friend, partner, or spouse can deepen your relationship.

Double Your Insight: Poses for Partners

Just as it's important to find wholeness and balance within, it's important to find it in all of your relationships. Practicing yoga with a fellow yogi can expand your awareness of the joys and sufferings of others and deepen your insight into the balance of relationships—with your fellow yogi and, ultimately, with all of humankind. It is also an excellent way to bond together, physically and spiritually, in a partnership. Try yoga with the man or woman you love and add a whole new dimension to your practice.

This set of poses can work with any pair—spouse, friend, partner, child.

Be a Mountain Range

A first and easy posture to try is Mountain pose, but because there are two of you, let's make it a mountain range. This is also a nice pose to do with the whole family! The more people involved, the longer your mountain range!

1. Face your partner, standing about two feet apart, and close your eyes. This distance is close enough to allow you to sense each other and to hold hands without arm strain, but far enough away to allow you to maintain a sense of your own space.

2. After you're both centered, hold hands. Take some time to become aware of your partner across from you (keep your eyes closed). Feel your partner's form and energy, then feel the energy flow between you as it traverses the bridge made from your joined hands.

3. Next, connect with the grounding energy of the earth. Feel how it pulls you toward its center. Feel your feet and legs connecting and becoming one with the earth.

4. Let the earth's energy move through your body, from toe to head and beyond. Through your joined hands, you can begin to sense the subtle energy of your physical forms and energy of the world around you.

5. **Continuing the Challenge:** For more than two people, stand side by side in Mountain pose, holding hands, and feet lined up. You can also stand with your legs about two feet apart so the side of each person's foot stands firmly against the side of the next person's foot.

Warrior 2 Pose for Two

Warrior pose will help you find balance with a partner. In the process, you'll both become stronger.

1. Stand with one of you in front (Partner A) and one behind (Partner B). Both perform the Warrior 2 pose (see Chapter 6). Once you are both in position, Partner A balances the extended arms and hands on top of the back of Partner B's extended arms, forming a chain of energy.

2. Partner B keeps Partner A's arms and hands at shoulder height. Partner B will expend more effort, but Partner A should keep the arms energized and strong rather than let them sag limply on Partner B's. Partner B should be supporting an energy flow, not a limp noodle.

3. Switch sides. Now Partner A holds Partner B's arms up. Breathe. Try to increase the length of time holding the pose. Encourage each other to hang in there. This pose is difficult and builds arm strength in addition to doubling the Warrior energy.

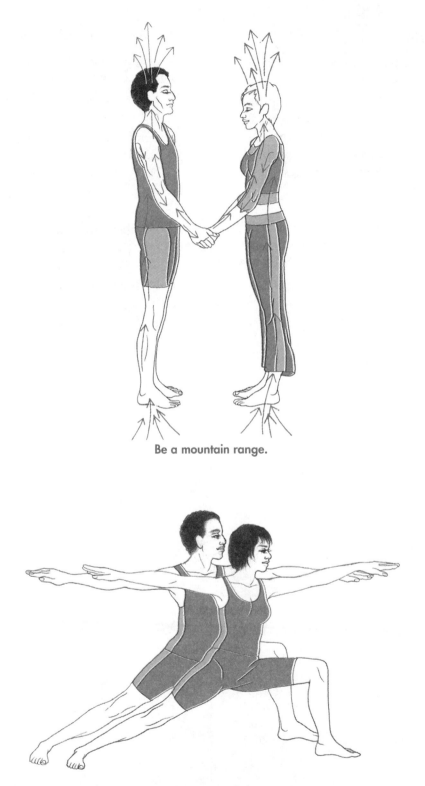

Be a mountain range.

Warrior 2 Pose for Two.

Stretch and Pull

Both partners receive a nice spine stretch in this pose for two.

1. Again, stand with one partner in front (Partner A) and one behind (Partner B). Partner B squats with heels on the floor. Partner A performs a forward bend, folding the torso forward at the hips. Partner A should be able to see Partner B between his or her legs.

2. Partner A reaches both hands between the legs, and Partner B grasps Partner A's wrists, pulling slightly to help Partner A stretch.

3. At the same time, Partner B bends down into a full squat, stretching the back.

4. Hold and take some breaths.

5. Switch places and do it again.

Lengthen Your Spines Together

Continue to lengthen the spine—maybe even grow an inch with this one!

1. Face each other, hold hands, then take a big step away from each other.

2. Bend at your hips, but don't clunk heads! Be sure to step far enough away from each other that you don't collide.

3. Bring your tailbones up and out. Take turns pulling gently on each other to lengthen your spines.

4. Then find a balance—pull—and both of you come down into a squat. Keep your heels on the ground. Stretch those spines.

5. Slowly come back up, balancing and stretching all the way back to standing.

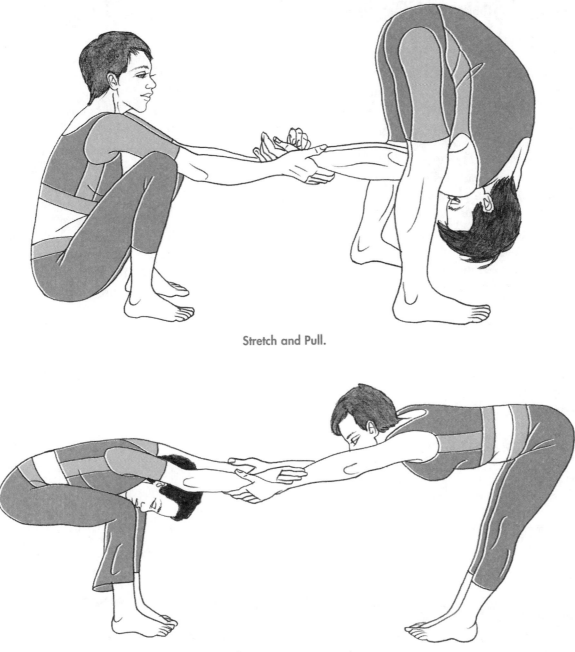

Stretch and Pull.

Lengthen Your Spines Together.

Sex and Spirituality: Poses for Couples

Practicing yoga with your significant other can deepen all aspects of your relationship, even your physical relationship. When practicing "couples yoga" with your partner, it's about more than simply holding positions—it's about connecting on a spiritual level. Truly connecting with your partner on a spiritual level is a much more blissful experience than physical connection void of any emotional or spiritual bond.

If you aren't used to connecting on this deep level, it can even be a little disconcerting. That's because souls are much more sensitive than bodies. It might not come easily right away, but it can be a goal you share with your partner as you do yoga together.

 A Yoga Minute

Mae West once said, "Sex is an emotion in motion." How true! One of the benefits of the fourth yama, brahmacharya (see Chapter 2), is that it teaches you to separate lust from a purer, spiritual connection. When you're fraught with emotional desire for the physical, you cannot perceive a deeper reality. Transcending intense emotions permits the spirit to manifest itself.

Prepare yourself for the possibility that problems might surface in your relationship. Your bodies can reflect your minds, so when you have difficulty with a double pose, look into what's wrong and see if you can't find what's happening on a deeper level. Working through the barriers in your physical partnership can reveal the barriers in your spiritual partnership. The lessons you learn are lessons in true love!

Here are some poses just for the two of you.

Massage Your Spines Together

This pose will help your partner connect to the muscles along the spine. A flexible spine equals a youthful body. Help your partner loosen up his or her spine.

1. Partner A sits in Child's pose (see Chapter 11).

2. Partner B stands behind Partner A and places a palm on either side of Partner A's spine at the lower back. Partner B gradually walks the hands up to the neck and back down to the lower back. Partner B keeps as much of the palm on Partner A's back as possible at all times, pressing gently. Don't press directly on the spine; stay on either side. Bend the knees, Partner B, if your back hurts.

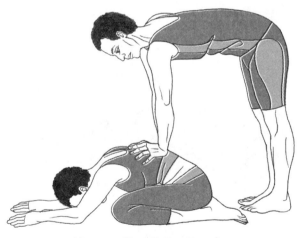

Massage Your Spines Together.

Forward Bend Together

This pose starts to look complicated, but it really isn't. It's only two poses in one. Partner B helps Partner A lengthen the spine by pushing down on Partner A's hipbone. Conversely, Partner A helps Partner B lengthen the hamstrings by pushing down on Partner B's heels.

1. Partner A gets into Child's pose with arms outstretched in front (see Chapter 11).

2. Partner B stands in front of Partner A. Partner A holds Partner B's ankles as Partner B assumes Downward Facing Dog (see Chapter 11) over the top of Partner A, placing the hands on either side of Partner A's hips, palms facing in.

3. Partner B helps Partner A lengthen the spine, while Partner A helps Partner B lengthen the hamstrings.

4. Hold as long as is comfortable, then switch positions.

Forward Bend and Backbend Together

Try this one with a partner who is about the same size as you are.

1. Partner A sits on the floor a few feet from a wall with the back to the wall and the feet in front and together. Bending at the waist, Partner A brings the chest toward the thighs. Bend your knees if needed.

2. Partner B lies on Partner A's back, facing up, and props the feet against the wall so that the feet are slightly higher than the head. Partner B's fingers can rest lightly on the ground on either side of Partner A's hips.

3. Hold for a while, then switch.

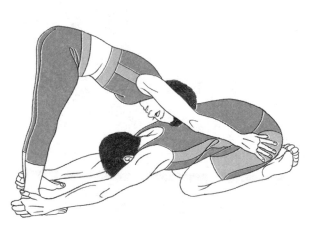

Forward Bend Together.

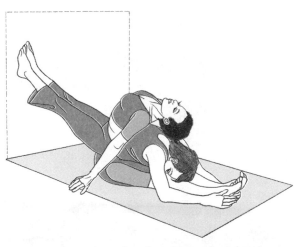

Forward Bend and Backbend Together.

Hero Pose for Two

Who says heroes can't come in pairs? This pose retains the tall, proud posture of Hero pose but lets two in on the fun.

1. Sit in Hero pose, back to back.

2. Link arms and pull gently to further expand the chest and breathing area.

3. As you both breathe, feel your spine and head stretching upward, and feel your partner doing the same thing.

4. Notice how deeply you are able to breathe together.

Boat Pose for Two

Boat Pose for Two helps calm the rocky waters and strengthens tummies, too.

1. Face each other so your hips are three to four feet apart. Both partners assume Boat pose (see Chapter 11).

2. Place your feet sole to sole, and grasp hands on the outsides of your legs. Now you look like a schooner!

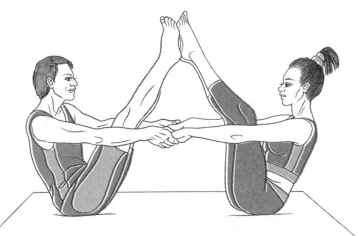

Boat Pose for Two.

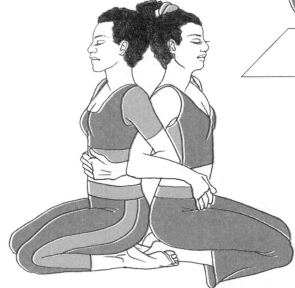

Hero Pose for Two with locked arms.

Candlesticks for Two

This energizing and supportive inversion brings two energies together in a vibrant flow. We call this modified shoulderstand Candlesticks for Two! You'll feel great after this pose, and more energetically linked to your partner. You can also do this pose in a triad or in a group of four. Just put your heads together and touch toes.

1. Lie down so the crowns of your heads are barely touching.

2. Gently raise your legs and hips, supporting your hips with your arms.

3. Bend your knees over your head and tilt back until you feel your partner's legs. Rest your lower legs against each other.

4. Hold until one or both of you are ready to come back down.

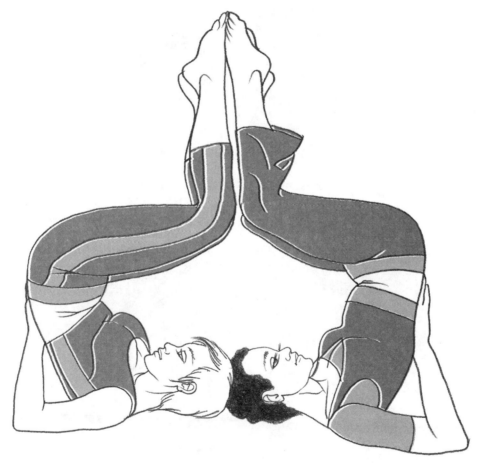

Candlesticks for Two.

Partner Tree

Balance the inverted Shoulderstand for two with this upright standing pose. This pose is a balance pose, yet the partnership makes it incredibly stable and grounding.

1. Stand side by side, shoulders touching or a couple inches apart.
2. Each partner bends outside knees and brings feet up.
3. Clasp each other's feet and bring opposite hands behind you. Hold opposite hands together.

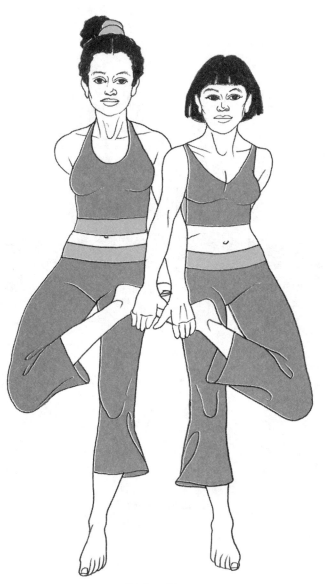

Partner Tree.

All in the Family

Finally, know that yoga can be a great way to bond with your family. Children of all ages—babies to teenagers—will benefit from yoga. Poses can be playful and fun for younger kids, pretending that they are an eagle or a boat or a tree. Teenagers take to yoga easily because of their natural flexibility. And just think how powerful it is to share the honor of the light in each of you—together. Namaste.

The Least You Need to Know

- Practicing yoga with a partner is fun and can deepen your relationship, making all aspects of your partnership—physical, emotional, and intellectual—more spiritual.
- Practicing yoga with a partner can help you stretch farther than you could alone.
- Yoga means union, coming together, yoking. So bring your partner along!
- Yoga honors the light within each and every family member.

In This Chapter

- What is beauty?
- How yoga can help you through PMS and menstruation
- Yoga for pregnant women and new mothers
- Yoga for menopause

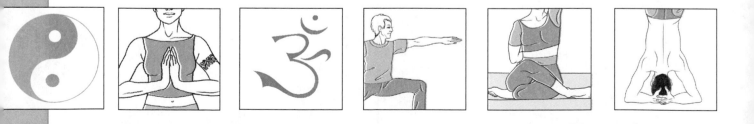

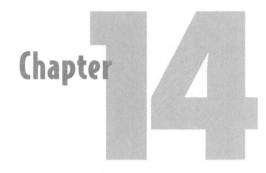

For Women Only

This chapter is for all you female yoginis out there! Being a woman means certain things biologically and certain things culturally, too. We experience menstruation as our first rite of passage into womanhood, many of us experience childbirth, and eventually we all experience menopause. We're also raised in a culture obsessed with beauty, youth, and the female body. Women have many unique challenges, and yoga can help with all of them by helping keep us fit, strong, clear-thinking, and joyful.

The Truth About Beauty

Beauty really isn't skin-deep. Beauty begins much deeper. In a superficial world, though, this deep truth gets lost, and many contemporary women have lost sight of their own inner and outer beauty. If you haven't found your inner self and aren't in touch with who you are, it's difficult to perceive your true beauty. Know that your inner beauty has nothing to do with your hair color or facial wrinkles or cellulite or breast size. These are transitory features of your soul's container. These aren't you.

The most important first step any woman can take in dealing with the issue of beauty is to practice ahimsa, or nonviolence. Nonviolent acceptance of yourself, not only physically but mentally and spiritually, is yoga's dictum. Don't commit violence to your body, either physically, by trying to force it to conform to some cultural ideal, or mentally, by hating it or obsessing over it. Remember that your body is a tool. Keep it well maintained so it doesn't interfere with the real you. Keep it clean, strong, and flexible, but also keep it in its place.

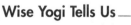

> **Wise Yogi Tells Us**
>
> When it comes to your body image, remember the yama of ahimsa, non-violence that we mentioned in Chapter 2. Not accepting your body as you are is a form of emotional violence, in which you are at odds with the body that is a gift to you.

The true you is much deeper, more complex, and more spectacular than your body. You are a manifestation of the universe. Finding yourself through yoga means finding the beautiful, spiritual you and bringing it out for everyone to see. Loving yourself means loving the universe, and loving the universe means loving yourself, because you're one and the same—you're both exquisitely radiant.

Managing PMS with Yoga

When you're suffering from premenstrual syndrome (PMS), you probably don't feel very radiant. PMS is a condition that affects a lot of women before the onset of their menstrual periods. Symptoms are as diverse as the women who experience them: overall discomfort, bloating, backache, headache, irritability, food cravings, depression, exaggerated emotions or sudden lack of emotion, acne, painful or swollen breasts, insomnia, fatigue, even uncharacteristically violent or suicidal behavior. Some women get emotional, uncomfortable, or hungrier, yet everyone is different, and each woman may experience different symptoms from month to month. Many women experience no symptoms at all.

Most women need extra calcium all month long, but many of us don't get the 1,000 mg per day we really need (1,500 mg per day if osteoporosis runs in your family). Recent studies show that increased calcium intake can dramatically relieve some of the uncomfortable symptoms of

PMS, so make sure that when it's that time of the month, you've "got milk" (or at least, calcium supplements!).

PMS commonly occurs during the week or two before the start of your period and can last until menstruation starts. You might notice a dramatic disappearance of symptoms, which can signal when menstruation is just about to begin (handy for the irregularly cycled among us). Symptoms are generally attributed to the production of hormones related to the menstrual cycle. You might not care about the cause so much as a good remedy when you're in the throes.

How can yoga help? Your hormone-wracked body will appreciate the familiar routine of the exercise. Triangle pose, sitting poses to open the hips, and twisting poses for lower back stiffness are all excellent for PMS. Although all the asanas activate the body, poses that stimulate the glandular and reproductive systems such as Cobra, Bow, and Bridge poses are especially good to practice during PMS.

> **Wise Yogi Tells Us**
>
> If you are feeling the symptoms of PMS, lie on your back with your buttocks against a wall. Put your legs up against the wall, separate them a bit, and lie there for a while—very relaxing.

Also, step up your pranayama practice. As your body sheds its uterine lining, support it by cleansing the rest of your body through pranayama (deep-breathing exercises). Pranayama also eases irritability, depression, and moodiness. Mantra work, too, can be of great benefit when your emotions are changing rapidly. The steady flow and vibration of a mantra soothes your nervous system and can help transform negative outbursts into outbursts of pure inspiration!

Evening primrose oil, dong quai, blessed thistle, cayenne, raspberry leaves, sarsaparilla, and Siberian ginseng are herbs known to help relieve symptoms of PMS such as bloating, pain, and depression. Look for these herbs in your local health food store. Check with your doctor first, though, particularly if you are taking other medication.

And no matter how bad PMS is, stress only makes it worse—just one more reason to keep practicing yoga! All the stress-reduction benefits of yoga can also help lessen the effects of PMS. Don't forget shavasana (the relaxation pose in Chapter 12)—do it as often as you can. When you are feeling physically or emotionally uncomfortable, you'll welcome shavasana's utterly relaxed state, especially when you get so relaxed that you don't even feel your body anymore!

Meditation, too, can be helpful when you are uncomfortable but in a good frame of mind. Meditation, including shavasana, can help you move beyond your physical body for a while and give you a break from your body's aches and pains.

Ouch!

PMS can literally be a big pain, and eating certain foods just before you expect PMS can make it worse. Try to avoid chocolate, caffeine, alcohol, excess salt, red meat, sugar, and overly processed foods, which seem to aggravate PMS symptoms in some women. Focus on calcium and fiber instead. A fresh apple and a glass of milk, anyone?

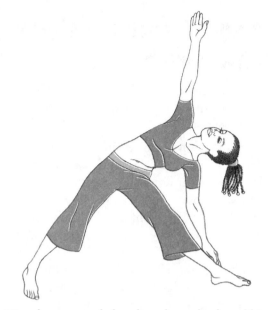

Triangle pose can help relieve lower back and hip pain associated with PMS.

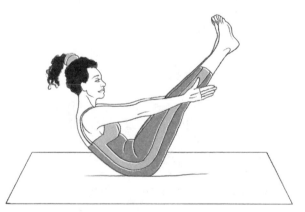

Boat pose can help relieve abdominal cramps associated with menstruation.

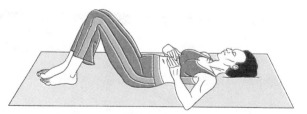

Stressed from PMS? Relax. Breathe deeply. Go with the flow (so to speak!).

Going Full Cycle: Celebrating Menstruation

Menstruation is a monthly marker of fertility and one of the few biologically imposed rituals we, as women, have.

Menstruation occurs in many women on a lunar schedule—a 28-day cycle—rather than a calendar month. For that reason and many more, women are linked in mythology to the moon. It might be helpful to you to notice the moon cycle for a few months, checking in with it nightly as it waxes and wanes. Start noticing its effect on you. How do you feel different during a full moon versus a new moon? Have you ever noticed that your menstrual cycle is in sync with the moon—either ovulating or menstruating with the full moon? Let what you notice carry over to a new reverence for your own body. (And check out our moon salutations in Chapter 16 for yoga's way of getting in touch with the moon.)

Incorporating yoga into your menstrual ritual is a nice way to make your monthly experience even more positive. You can do most yoga poses you normally do, but you might enjoy creating a special yoga routine for the week of your menstrual period. Listen to your body especially well during this sensitive time, and enjoy a nice, relaxing rest on the floor with your legs and feet up against the wall.

You might use the following pose, but you also might want to experiment with Triangle, Cobra, Bow (great for cramps if you're up to it, and very energizing), Wheel (also great for cramps), Bridge, Butterfly, Lotus, and Moon Salutation. Also remember that an extra-long shavasana is the perfect way to end your yoga practice during your menstrual cycle.

1. Sit in Hero, Butterfly, or Lotus pose. Place a few pillows stacked on top of each other directly behind you.

2. Lie back on top of the pillows. Extend your arms over your head. This position opens the fourth chakra and is also a good variation to perform during pregnancy.

Wise Yogi Tells Us

Rather than fighting gravity, yoga makes a friend of gravity. So during those times when we want to encourage movement out of the body, such as during menstruation, it's counterproductive to work against gravity by practicing inversions like the Headstand or the Plough. Thank gravity for helping your body with its monthly "out with the old, in with the new" process and do not overly extend inversions during this time.

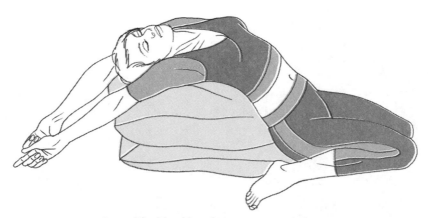

A modified backbend eases menstruation.

So You're Having a Baby!

Pregnancy yoga is slightly different than regular yoga, and perhaps even more wonderful. Yoga helps you develop a greater awareness of your body so you can respond better to your body's subtle signals when you are doing too much or you really need an infusion of green vegetables. Because yoga gets you moving, you'll be in better shape for childbirth. Recovery and getting back to your prepregnancy shape will be easier, too.

Taking a prenatal yoga class can be quite beneficial—and fun, too. You'll meet other pregnant yoginis, and you'll get qualified instruction on the safest and most beneficial yoga poses. Plus, in the last month or two when your baby is getting big, he or she may be able to move more freely as you open your body in a stretch.

A few caveats first, however. Take these precautions when practicing pregnancy yoga:

- Tell your doctor you are practicing yoga, and get permission for all poses you plan on practicing. If your doctor isn't familiar with yoga, bring pictures of the poses you'd like to do.
- Avoid extreme stretching positions and any position that puts pressure on or contracts your uterus. Skull Shining Breath might be too jarring for your baby, and full forward bends will probably be uncomfortable for you and baby, too. Be careful also with spinal twists. Try to focus on the upper part of the spine and do not over twist the mid and lower parts of your spine.
- Avoid full backbends such as Wheel pose and full forward bends such as Standing Head to Knees—maintain that abdominal space.
- Keep standing poses to a minimum, and never jump into them.

- Remember that your center of balance is completely different than it was before you were pregnant. Be careful doing balance poses.
- Don't lie on your stomach for any pose.
- After the twentieth week, don't lie on your back for any pose. The weight of the baby can hinder your blood flow. (More than likely, you will find this so uncomfortable that you won't want to do it, anyway.)

The following poses are only suggestions. If any pose feels uncomfortable or strenuous, stop at once. If you experience dizziness, sudden swelling, extreme shortness of breath, or vaginal bleeding, see your doctor immediately. Your best approach to these postures is to listen to your body and not take it where it doesn't want to go.

- **Mountain pose.** Focus on tilting your lower back in to prevent the weight of the baby from pressing against your lumbar. Bend your knees slightly and place your hands on top of your knees. Tighten your thigh muscles and watch your kneecaps lift upward. Straighten your legs and try to lift your kneecaps.
- **Corpse pose.** After your twentieth week, practice shavasana lying on your left side. A pillow for your head and pillows between your knees can take pressure off your neck, lower back, and hips.
- **Hero pose.** Sitting in Hero pose helps reduce swelling in your ankles, reduces fatigue, and improves circulation in your legs. Place a stack of pillows behind you and lean back. Bring your hands alongside your body to push yourself back up.
- **Child's pose.** Support your body with a stack of pillows placed between your knees, or stand on your knees and cross your arms over the back of a chair and lean forward. You might also want a pillow or blanket under your knees.

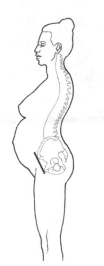

The added weight of pregnancy can create a condition called lordosis, a swayback effect. Practice Mountain pose and concentrate on maintaining the proper spinal and pelvic alignment.

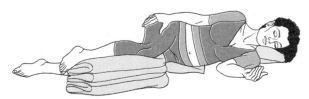

After the twentieth week of pregnancy, practice shavasana by lying on your left side.

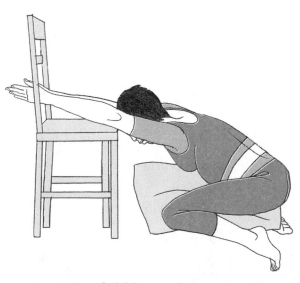

A variation of Child's pose during pregnancy.

◆ **Simple hamstring stretches.** Hamstring stretches relieve pressure on your lower back. Be gentle when you stretch.

◆ **Twisting poses.** *Always do these gently when pregnant!* When not pregnant, your focus should be on twisting your entire spine. During pregnancy, however, most of your twisting will be in your neck, shoulders, and head. Lift your spine as you inhale, and twist as you exhale.

Ouch!

At the first sign of leg cramps (common in pregnancy), draw your toes upward and push out your heel. Practice this movement so you can be ready to perform it in a split second when a leg cramp wakes you up in the middle of the night.

◆ **Warrior 2 or Side Angle Stretch, using a chair for support.** Try these poses seated on the center of a chair. The variation illustrated is more freeing and takes the weight off your legs.

◆ **Downward Facing Dog, using a chair for support.** What a wonderful stretch and release for your spine! Holding on to the chair takes some of the pressure off your legs in this pose. You'll feel freer, and so will your little passenger.

◆ **Butterfly pose.** This pose can help you relax, open your hips, and prepare for labor. If your hip joints are tight, sit supported with a pillow under each knee. Hold the position only as long as it is comfortable. Move into an Easy pose and rest if you need to.

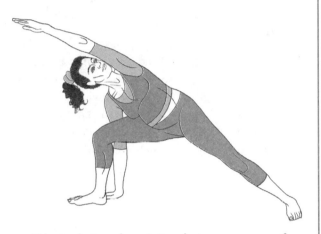

Side Angle Stretch variation during pregnancy. If you need more support, do this pose with a straight-backed chair and be sure you are balanced firmly on the seat to give you more stability.

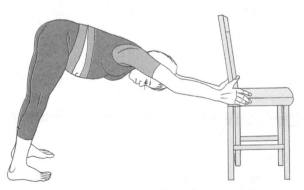

Downward Facing Dog variation during pregnancy. If you don't have a steady, firm chair to use, place your hands against a wall and stretch this way.

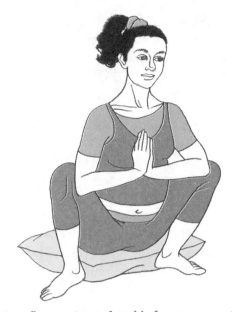

If Butterfly pose is comfortable for you, you might want to try this more advanced squatting pose. Stack the pillows as high on the floor as you need to, to reduce stress on your joints and muscles. When you are ready, return to a seated meditative position and breathe deeply and fully.

New Mama Yoga

Maybe before you had your baby, you thought about doing yoga to get back in shape, but now you are home with your little bundle of joy, and you're incredulous that you could have ever thought you would have time for yoga. You don't even have time to sleep!

But practicing yoga now is important because you need the energy. Filling your body with prana through breathing exercises and 10 minutes daily in shavasana will recharge you and make the little sleep you do get more effective in restoring you. Your body also needs all its resources to heal itself after childbirth.

You probably need some mental maintenance, too. Your hormones might be making you extra emotional after childbirth. Add to that the fact that your entire life has changed and will never be the same. Pile on top of that the fact that your jeans look hopelessly small, and even though you aren't pregnant anymore, all you might be able to wear are your old maternity clothes. Remember that it takes time to adjust to any major life change. It will also take your body time to readjust to a nonpregnant state. Be patient. Be kind to yourself. It took you nine months to get to childbirth, so give yourself nine months to get back. You have just accomplished something magnificent, and it has changed you. Accept the change lovingly and with joy.

Give yourself time to practice yoga each day, either when your baby is sleeping or when your partner, a family member, or a friend can care for the baby. Consider it pampering time and a well-deserved reward.

With your doctor's approval, you can usually start gentle yoga poses two weeks after delivery (more if you had a cesarean section). Hold off on inverted poses for at least six weeks.

All women have postnatal bleeding for a few weeks after pregnancy. Watch this flow for signs that you're going too fast. If the bleeding gets heavier or brighter red, you need to slow down and give your doctor a call. Start with just a few poses, and gradually work back to your regular routine as your body lets you know it's ready.

Wise Yogi Tells Us

A high-sugar diet will make you feel tired anytime, but especially in the early weeks after childbirth. Sure, you deserve a treat now and then, but a diet based on whole grain foods like whole wheat bread and brown rice, sufficient iron (best sources are dark, leafy greens, wheat germ, and meat), and lots of vegetables is the best diet to combat fatigue.

The most beneficial pose for you right now is shavasana, which you can even do on the day you give birth. Shavasana can help ease labor pains, help you recoup your energy before all that pushing, and also help you relax after the whole process is finished and you have a sleeping baby on your chest.

Any chance you get, take some deep breaths and practice these revitalizing poses. You'll handle all your new challenges with greater inner strength and energy. The following poses are also wonderful for a gentle postpregnancy routine:

◆ **Mountain pose.** Take some time to stand in Mountain pose, and notice how your center of gravity has shifted yet again. Let tadasana help you reacquaint yourself with your newly autonomous body.

◆ **Child's pose.** Let yourself be the child for a few minutes each day.

◆ **Lying Down Spinal Twist.** Let your body relax for long periods of time in this pose to make up for all the spinal twisting you needed to forego during pregnancy. Relax and enjoy!

The postpartum (the period after childbirth) time is a good time to read the *Yoga Sutras* or other yoga texts. Keep them on a bedside or end table to read while nursing your baby or while baby is sleeping … or read them out loud to your baby to help quiet her with the sound of your voice and get her started on her yoga journey at the outset!

Easing Through Menopause

Menopause is the time of life when a woman stops ovulating. Although the age at which it occurs varies greatly, it commonly occurs around age 50. Yet menopause means much more to women than this simple biological definition. The thought of menopause is daunting to many, and it's no wonder! Our culture puts so much emphasis on youth and beauty, especially for women, that aging is difficult.

Far from being the end of life, menopause signals a period of life during which spiritual growth can soar. Women who have passed through menopause often feel stronger, more in charge of their lives, and more intimately acquainted with their souls than ever before. Age brings wisdom, and once a woman is no longer a childbearer, her body can focus on its own journey. Increasing numbers of strong, vibrant, amazing older women have become important figures in our culture. Look to these women as examples for your own life. This next stage of your journey may be the most thrilling yet. It's certainly full of possibilities.

But first, you have to get through the menopause, and that isn't always pleasant. A hot flash is still a hot flash (you could call it a recharge!). Other symptoms of decreased estrogen levels are dizziness, depression, heart palpitations, decreased sex drive, and shortness of breath.

Yoga balances the endocrine system and can ease the difficult transition by stabilizing hormone levels. Inverted postures are particularly helpful for hot flashes, because they cool the body and fill it with prana. All the inversions will make you feel more vital because they replenish and rejuvenate your body. However, don't do inversions if you have high blood pressure.

Pranayama, too, is cooling to the body.

As you work through menopause, incorporate these postures into your yoga routine:

- **Headstand and other inversions, like Shoulderstand and Plough.** If you've never mastered Headstand, now's the time to try. Headstand might reduce your hot flashes.

- **Downward Facing Dog and other forward-bending postures, such as Standing Head to Knees and Yoga Mudra.** These forward-bending poses help you focus inwardly, an important process right now. Instead of shunning your body or feeling that it has betrayed you, embrace it, get to know it all over again, and let it work for you, leading you to a higher spiritual plane.

- **Sun Salutation.** Celebrate how your body has moved beyond moonlike cycles and catapulted like a rocket on toward the sun. Make the sun your newest ally. If you're up to it, start rising at dawn to practice yoga. Notice how, although the earth moves and turns and changes, the sun burns steadily and luminously in the center of our solar system. Meditate on how your body has become sunlike and strong, glowing with newfound steadiness and bliss.

- **Any weight-bearing postures and activities.** A drop in your estrogen level can cause you to lose bone mass, but you can easily counter this by exercising your bones. Postures that put stress on your bones such as inversions, standing postures, and Downward Facing Dog all increase bone mass. Light weightlifting is great for your bones and so is walking. Take a walk in the fresh air every day to keep your bones strong, your lungs full, and your heart light.

◆ **Legs on Wall.** Place a folded blanket or pillows about nine inches high against a wall. Support your lower and mid-back on the blanket, stretch your legs up the wall, and let your shoulder blades and head rest on the floor. Rest in this pose for 10 minutes with your eyes closed; focus on your breathing. This pose is cooling and therapeutic for any pelvic or abdominal problems.

◆ **Meditation.** Start regular meditation. You're in an excellent time of life to begin. You have a better sense of yourself than ever before. Take advantage of your wisdom and experience, and reap the benefits of meditation.

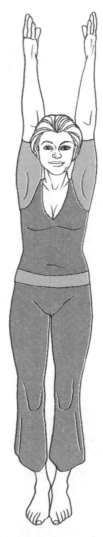

Practice breathing in Mountain pose. Inhale and lift your arms over your head. Exhale and bring your arms and hands down into Prayer pose. Return to Mountain and repeat. Yoga breathing helps lower blood pressure and reduce stress in mind and body.

Celebrate Your Femininity

No matter what stage of life you're in, yoga can help you ease through the physical and mental challenges. Yoga can deepen your experience of these passages, sharpen your mental acuity, and enrich your emotional and spiritual life.

The Least You Need to Know

◆ Beauty has nothing to do with your physical appearance. If you care for your body and radiate inner bliss, you'll be beautiful.

◆ Yoga can help reduce symptoms of PMS and menstruation.

◆ Yoga can be tailored to accommodate pregnancy and new motherhood.

◆ Yoga can ease the transition of menopause.

In This Chapter

- ◆ Yoga for your aching back and other pains
- ◆ Yoga for fatigue
- ◆ Warding off colds and flu
- ◆ Yoga for relief from chronic illnesses

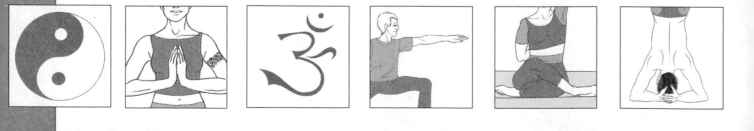

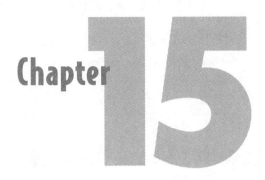

Yoga Eases Aches and Pains

No matter how much we appreciate our bodies, they don't always function perfectly. We get the flu bug that's going around or suffer from insomnia, back pain, or indigestion. And sometimes, despite our best efforts, we end up with chronic conditions.

But the yogi has a few extra tricks to hold pain, discomfort, and illness at bay. Read on for how to help prevent, relieve, and sometimes even heal your health problems.

Yoga Activates Healing

The healthy yogi knows the body has its own natural healing mechanisms and uses yoga to promote the optimum conditions for warding off aches and pains, illnesses, and diseases. The key is balance between body, mind, and spirit and the proper amount of pranayama. By practicing right living—avoiding too much high-sugar food, caffeine, tobacco, or alcohol, for instance—yogis minimize the ways these things detract from our vitality, or *svasthya*. Yoga takes a holistic approach to health.

Svasthya (*SVAH-sthyah*) is the Sanskrit word for "health," from *sva-stha*, which means "one's own state." Roga (*ROH-gah*) means "sickness," and vyadhi (*VYAH-dee*) means "disease."

Yoga for Those Nagging Complaints

Yoga is good therapy for the minor health problems that plague you. You'll probably find that with regular, consistent yoga practice, you'll suffer less often from minor complaints. If they do arise, however, try a few appropriate yoga asanas and stick with your yoga rules for living (yamas and niyamas) for effective relief.

A Yoga Minute

Back pain sufferers might need more calcium and magnesium. Great sources are milk, yogurt, cheese, dark leafy greens like collard greens and kale, calcium-fortified orange juice, almonds, calcium-fortified tofu, broccoli, wheat bran, wheat germ, whole wheat flour, calcium-fortified cereal, dried beans, peanut butter, and dried apricots.

Oh, My Aching Back ...

Because we all walk around upright, our backs are bound to suffer. Our poor spines carry all that weight around and are continually jarred by the pounding of our feet, not to mention twisted and contorted by less-than-perfect postures. Weak stomach muscles are a common cause of back pain.

Injury to a disc or vertebrae can cause back pain. Yoga can help in these cases. If you suffer from back pain, include the following exercises, which strengthen the stomach and/or tone the spine, in your yoga routine:

- ◆ Cobra pose (Chapter 7)
- ◆ Single Leg Lifts (Chapter 8)
- ◆ Boat pose (Chapter 11)

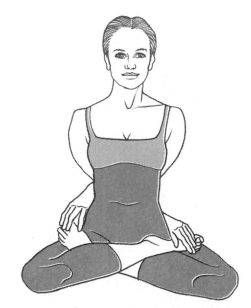

Yoga poses such as Bound Lotus can help you protect against bone and muscle loss, prevent the compression fractures common with osteoporosis, and encourage good posture as you age.

Oh, My Aching Head ...

All kinds of things cause headaches—foods, air pollution, allergies, sinus problems, eyestrain, or stress, for starters. Eliminate the suspected culprits, such as caffeine or certain foods. Naturally, if your headaches are severe or your headache patterns change, see a doctor. For occasional, irregular headaches, however, your best bet might be to step up your yoga practice.

For headache relief, try the following:

◆ Try pranayama breathing techniques (Chapter 10).

◆ Gently rotate and flex your neck and toes.

◆ Practice inverted postures where your head is lower than your heart. Inverted postures increase the flow of oxygen to the brain, but don't try these if you have high blood pressure.

◆ Take a tip from reflexology, a healing art that uses targeted foot massage to reduce pain and induce healing. Pull on your big toe gently, straight from its socket, and hold the pull.

Why Am I So Tired?

Fatigue is a common problem in our over-extended and fast-paced lives. Sometimes we simply wear ourselves out! Fatigue can also be caused by stress and extreme mental exertion, such as when you've been studying excessively, or when you're bothered by an emotional problem such as depression or anxiety. A good holistic health-care practitioner or therapist might be able to help you discover the under-lying cause of your fatigue. Stress on your endocrine system, the system that produces hormones, can cause fatigue. If you notice unusual fatigue, even when you've gotten enough sleep, consult a physician.

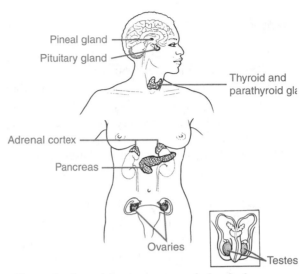

The endocrine system is a group of glands that man-ufacture hormones. Many yoga poses compress and stimulate these glands.

Wise Yogi Tells Us

A few lifestyle modifications could be the answer to eliminating fatigue in your life. Try the following:

◆ Getting off caffeine ASAP!

◆ Not eating anything sweet before noon.

◆ Eating a low-fat diet. Too much fat slows you down and wears you out.

◆ Maintaining a positive attitude. Don't sweat the small stuff!

◆ Lifting your own weight in yoga poses.

For occasional bouts of fatigue during the day, a 20-minute power nap can work wonders. If you aren't in a position to take a nap, try the following:

◆ Practice shavasana, or Corpse pose, for five minutes. (Chapter 12)

◆ Do deep-breathing exercises to replenish your prana.

◆ Do backbends to help energize you. (Chapter 7)

Why Can't I Sleep?

Stress is a common factor with insomnia, too. How can you sleep when your mind is buzzing with the worries of the day? If you have trouble getting to sleep, you probably already know to lay off the caffeine, especially in the evening, and not to eat a whole pepperoni pizza at midnight. But if your busy mind is keeping you up at night, try the following:

◆ Meditate. Evening meditation can calm and still your mind, making sleep easier. Many wise yogis sit in Full Lotus in meditation so that if—or when—they fall asleep, they won't fall over!

◆ Shavasana is as good for insomnia as it is for fatigue. If you are uncomfortable lying flat on the floor due to lower back or joint pain, place a pillow or rolled blanket under your knees and another under your head and neck for support when practicing yoga's shavasana pose (Chapter 12).

◆ Forward bends quiet the body and mind (Chapter 11).

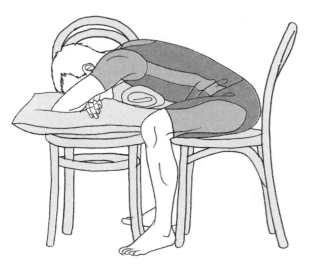

Forward bends are calming and can help induce sleep. This refreshing supported Child's pose stretch can help you relax.

◆ To help you get to sleep, take a warm bath before bed, and don't eat for at least three hours.

◆ Lavender oil in your bath or dried lavender stuffed in your pillowcase can help soothe you to sleep.

Breathing Clear: Yoga and Colds

Use pranayama to keep your breathing passages clear when you have a cold. If you are too congested to breathe through your nose, sit with your head over a bowl of hot water and a towel draped over your head. Poses that open up the chest can help: Bow, Fish, or Cobra (Chapter 7). If you have nasal congestion, try using a neti pot. A neti pot is a pot specifically tailored to the nose! A mixture of saline solution is poured into one nostril and comes out the other nostril with the appropriate tilt of the head.

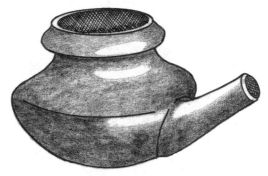

Neti pots are used to clear sinuses and for allergy sufferers.

Eyestrain Drain

Working at a computer or poring over paperwork all day can really strain your eyes. Yoga has many balancing exercises to help your eyes focus far away when they've been focused too close for too long, or to exercise and stretch the tiny muscles of your eye when they've been fixed in one place for too long (like that computer monitor). Try focusing on your thumb held at arm's length and following it up, down, right, left, and in clockwise and counterclockwise circles.

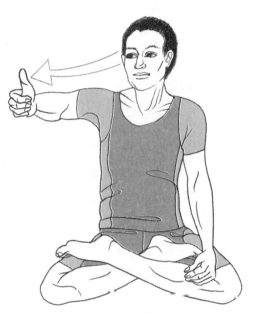

Follow your thumb up, down, right, left, and in circles to relieve eyestrain.

Digesting It All

Yoga helps with digestion, relieving gas, heartburn, and constipation, among other things. It keeps everything running smoothly. Remember, too, that your digestive success depends on not just what you eat, but how you eat. Eat your food slowly, savoring the flavors and textures. Rush it, and you'll likely end up with indigestion.

Sthala Basti (Ground Colon Cleansing): Elimination = Illumination!

Let's start at the bottom. This ritual helps relieve gas and keeps the bowels moving smoothly. It also improves digestion and gives your body a lighter feel.

Sit with your legs stretched out in front of you. Grab your big toes, right toe with your right hand, left toe with your left hand. Bend forward, bringing your head toward your knees just a little, so it feels comfortable. Relax your abdominal muscles, then churn them up and down. While churning your muscles, keep your gluteal muscles tight. Be very careful not to push yourself too hard. This ritual should feel comfortable. Be sure to practice this ritual on an empty stomach.

Tummy Toner

Yoga sequences that move the digestive area through compression and stretching are good for improving digestion. These yoga poses also help:

◆ Shavasana (Chapter 12).
◆ Fish pose (Chapter 7), which lengthens the abdomen, followed by Child's pose (Chapter 11), which compresses the abdomen
◆ Lightning Bolt pose (Chapter 6).
◆ Sun Salutation (Chapter 16).

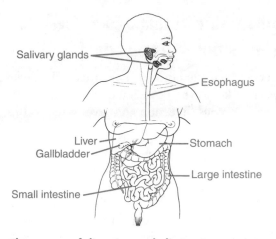

Salivary glands

Esophagus

Liver

Gallbladder

Stomach

Small intestine

Large intestine

The organs of digestion and elimination are compressed by forward-bending yoga poses, while back bends give these systems space or flexibility. Both contraction and flexibility are needed for healthy functioning.

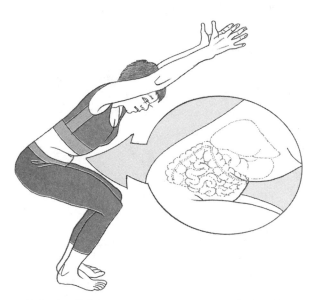

Lightning Bolt pose compresses organs of digestion and elimination to help stimulate and balance these important systems of the body.

Ouch!

This book is meant to complement, not replace, your doctor! If you are sick, injured, or suffer chronic pain, seek medical attention from a licensed medical professional. Tell your doctor you'd like to make yoga a part of your ongoing treatment plan.

Arthritis

Many people decrease activity because of arthritis pain, but yoga offers a way to keep your joints mobile, which keeps them limber and clean. Yoga encourages you to keep moving—but gently. Yoga can be a great help for arthritis and other forms of chronic joint pain, including TMJ (temporal mandibular joint), tennis elbow, and carpal tunnel syndrome.

Of course, it's important not to push yourself beyond what your body can do. Don't exercise joints that are inflamed.

- Vinyasana routines (Chapter 16), such as a slow Sun Salutation, are excellent for maintaining your mobility.

- Try self-massage to bring warmth and circulation to painful areas.

- Pranayama increases your circulation and helps with pain.

Asthma, Allergies, and Respiratory Problems

When your breath is disturbed, your prana delivery system is disturbed, and that's a big deal. You don't want to mess with the life force! But seriously, if you suffer from asthma, allergies, or other respiratory problems, try the following to keep your breath flowing freely:

◆ Practice poses that open and stretch the chest: Tree, Warrior (Chapter 6), Fish, Bow, and Cobra poses (Chapter 7). These poses give your lungs an extra deep stretch to encourage extra deep breaths.

◆ Two deep breaths while holding a pose are better than 10 shallow breaths.

Yoga and Your Healing

Illness, disease, and pain don't have to keep you from a fulfilling yoga practice. With your doctor's and yoga teacher's guidance, progress at a pace that is right for you and let yoga help your body help itself.

The Least You Need to Know

◆ Many things can cause or encourage illness or injury. Balancing the physical *and* energetic systems are essential in the overall healing journey.

◆ Don't blame yourself for getting sick or injured. Instead, focus on loving yourself and letting your body activate its natural processes for healing.

◆ The regular practice of yoga asanas and pranayama exercises is a great way to prevent health problems and to help your body heal itself when problems occur.

◆ Yoga can help with your minor health complaints, such as colds, minor back pain, and fatigue.

In This Part

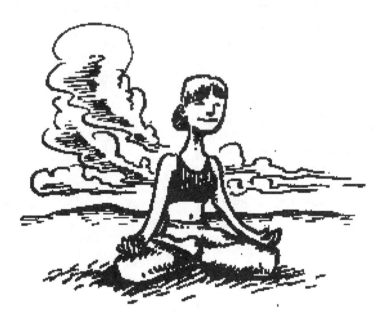

Part **5**

Yoga Sessions

Now, let's put it all together. We'll start with vinyasana, a method of yoga that strings poses together in a sequence, emphasizing deep breathing, to create an active, flowing routine. You'll learn how to make your routine into a cardiovascular workout, and you'll find out about Sun Salutations … and Moon Salutations, too!

Next, we'll give you some targeted and fully illustrated sessions to fit into your day. Whether you have 5 minutes, 15 minutes, half an hour, or a full hour for yoga, we've got a sequence of poses that will fit into your life.

In This Chapter

- Yoga's Sun Salutation

- Yoga's Moon Salutation

- Combining postures in a sequence of motion

- How to create your own flow—move and groove

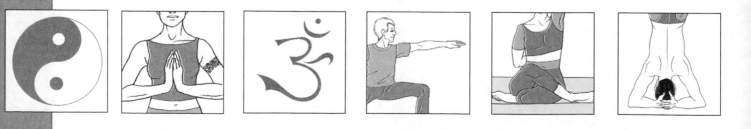

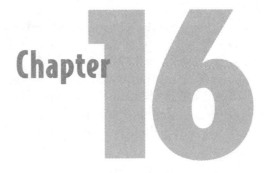

Chapter 16

Vinyasana: Moving with the Sun and the Moon

You're probably convinced by now that yoga can be tough and challenging to your strength and flexibility. But what about working up a *real* sweat? That's where vinyasana (*vin-YAH-sah-nah*) comes in! Vinyasana combines a series of yoga postures into a long, fluid, unified movement. Poses are held within a vinyasana, but the difference is that when you come out of one posture, you flow immediately into another posture. The right flow will give you a great workout, in addition to improving your balance, grace, speed, strength, and agility.

Finding Your Rhythm

Continuous-flow sequences of yoga postures can be an invigorating cardiovascular workout. Repeating a series of postures in quick succession takes stamina and good lung capacity. A more slowly executed series of poses is also challenging, allowing you to enter each pose fully and deliberately while still engaging in continuous movement. Whatever the pace, a vinyasana flows in a moving meditation. Let the rhythm of your body and your breath move you to new levels of bodymind awareness.

Breath Sets the Beat

Breath is extremely important in a vinyasana. Connecting posture to posture and movement to movement is more than just moving muscles. Every movement and every position of a vinyasana has an equivalent breath: an inhale, an exhale, or a hold. A good general guideline is to exhale when going into forward bends and inhale when going into backward bends.

The right breathwork in a vinyasana can make or break the flow of a series. Before you begin your vinyasana, determine your pace and your intention. For instance, maybe you decide to do the Sun Salutation in a slow and languid way this morning to warm you up. Let your breathing reflect this intention. Inhale and exhale deeply with each movement of this vinyasana. Perhaps you do it again this afternoon, but this time at a quicker, more energized pace. Again, let your breathing reflect your intention. Breathe to the rhythm of your movements so your breath and your body work together.

> **Wise Yogi Tells Us**
>
> When you set your intention ahead of time, you'll be in a better frame of mind to notice and monitor your progress as you go. Are you revving up too much, when you had intended to go slow? Are you lagging behind when you had intended to keep an upbeat pace?

Let your mind work with your body, as they become one, using your breath as a monitor. If you can't breathe slowly enough, deepen your breath or allow for more than one breath in a position. If you can't keep up, slow the pace. Let your breath work for you. It will tell you when you are pushing yourself too hard.

Always remember to breathe with your entire body during a vinyasana. Inhale fully, and exhale completely. Let the movements—the contractions and expansions, the bends and arches, twists and stretches—help your lungs and the muscles in your thoracic cavity draw breath in and push it out. Feel the breath traveling from your toes to your fingertips, your heels to your head. Let the breath be as integral to the movement as your physical body.

Bodymind in Motion

Just as your breath works for you during a vinyasana, so does your mind. More than your muscles are moving here! Your mind is to be equally engaged in the movement from pose to pose.

Making a purposeful effort to concentrate on the way your body feels and moves during a vinyasana is an excellent way to cultivate mindfulness. The vinyasana becomes a sort of meditation when practiced with this kind of intense focus. Let your moving body and flowing breath be the center of your meditation. Observe yourself from the inside out. Let your mind become the movement, let the movement become your body, let your body connect back to your mind in a complete circle.

You are one fully integrated, fully functioning yogi—so let's go with the flow!

Warming Up with Uttanatavasan: Leg Lifts

Uttanatavasan (*ooh-TAHN-ah-tah-VAH-sahn*), or Leg Lifts, prepare you to make the more fluid movements of a full vinyasana. Leg Lifts strengthen your stomach, which in turn supports your lower back. The deeper your breathing during this movement, the easier and smoother your vinyasana will become.

Be careful not to use momentum to swing your legs up during Leg Lifts. Keep your movements slow and complete to build your strength, touching the ground and pausing before each lift. Don't separate your feet or bend your knees when you come down. If your back hurts, keep one knee bent, foot on the floor, but keep the other leg straight.

A Yoga Minute

Regular practice of Leg Lifts can help alleviate lower back pain. A majority of Americans over age 40 suffer from it.

Single Leg Lift

Leg Lifts strengthen and tone the abdomen. A strong abdominal area makes for a strong lower back, giving stability for the muscles there.

1. Lie on your back. Bend your left leg a little and press your lower back toward the floor slightly to avoid lower back strain.

2. Inhale as you straighten your right leg and lift it. When your leg is perpendicular to the floor, push your heel out.

3. Exhale and slowly lower your leg back down.

4. Repeat this movement on the same side, connecting each repetition with breath: inhale as your leg goes up, exhale as your leg goes down.

5. Do three or four repetitions, then switch to your left leg.

Wise Yogi Tells Us

While flowing through a Single Leg Lift, cup your hands over your ears and listen intently to your breath as it connects movement to movement. Is it smooth? Rocky? Does it sound like the ocean? The wind in the trees? Link the rhythm of your breath to the movements of your muscles. Notice everything. Be mindful. Close your eyes. Internalize.

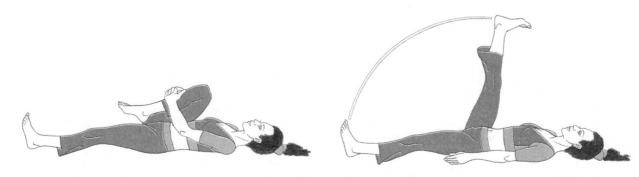

Single Leg Lift.

Double Leg Lift

Double the Leg Lift, double the strength! This movement requires stronger abdominal strength. Single Leg Lifts help build up this strength. Once your abs are strong, it's time to continue the challenge with both legs. Your back will love you for it, too.

1. Begin the Double Leg Lift with your palms facing downward and tucked under your tailbone to keep your lower back from rising off the floor. Straighten your arms out under you. If you have long arms, they might go past your tailbone, which is fine.

2. Slowly inhale as you bring both legs straight up while you contract your abdominal muscles, pulling them in toward the floor to further support your lower back. Keep your feet flexed and your heels pushed out.

3. Exhale as you bring both legs straight down, keeping your abdominals firmly contracted. Tuck in your chin so your neck does not overarch back.

4. Do as many lifts as you can, inhaling as your legs go up, exhaling as your legs come down. Move slowly. Then rest.

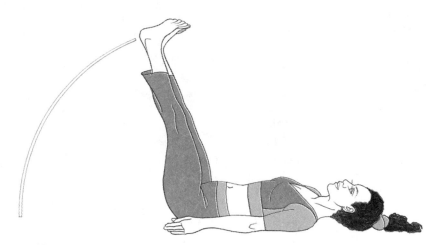

Double Leg Lift. Extend long through your fingertips, as you see in the illustration, and then place your hands palm down on the floor.

Sun Salutations

The sun is the center of our solar system, providing energy and warmth to our planet. This vinyasana is a devotional to the sun. Surya Namaskara (*SOOR-yah nah-mahs-KAH-rah*) offers thanks and greetings to the sun, and although it can be performed any time, it is particularly appropriate and wonderful when performed outdoors at sunrise, facing east. *Surya* means "sun," and *namaskara* literally means "taking a bow."

Sun Salutation energizes, strengthens, and tones all the major muscles and organs in your body.

Warming Up for the Sun: Banarasana

Banarasana (*bah-nah-RAH-sah-nah*), or Lunge pose, is used within Sun Salutation. Many people find it challenging, so it's good to first practice the pose on its own.

1. Stand in Mountain pose with your feet together, hands hanging down. Breathe.

2. Exhale and bend forward into Standing Head to Knees pose. Bend your knees if necessary to put your palms on the floor on both sides of your feet.

3. Inhale, and as you exhale, step one foot back behind you into what is commonly called a runner's lunge. Keep your chest forward and your head lifted.

4. Release your foot so the top of your foot is flat on the floor and drop your hips to try to make the line from your neck to your knee a straight line, diagonal with the floor. (It helps to do this in front of a mirror to check for the proper alignment.) Keep your palms flat on the floor so your fingers line up with your toes.

5. Hold for several moments, then draw your back foot back next to your other foot as you raise your hips, coming back into Standing Forward Bend.

6. Roll back up into Mountain pose.

7. Repeat with the other leg.

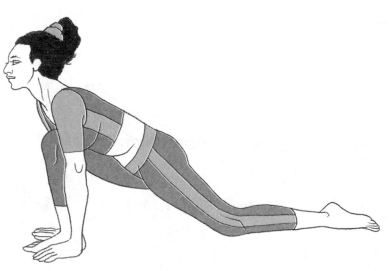

Lunge pose.

Surya Namaskara: Sun Salutation

This series of poses make up the classic Sun Salutation series, though there are many variations.

1. Mountain pose. Begin in Mountain pose with your hands in namaste, or prayer position. Center yourself and concentrate on a devotional attitude toward the sun.

2. Arms Extended. Inhale. Raise your arms up over your head and tilt them slightly back, as if you were encompassing the sun with love.

3. Standing Forward Bend. Exhale. Bring your hands straight down to the floor. Bend your knees to protect your lower back. Eventually, you may straighten your legs. Bring your palms alongside your feet. This position is a symbol of thanking the earth, where our feet are firmly planted.

4. Lunge. Keeping your hands down, inhale and step your left foot back behind you. Stay low to the ground and look up. This represents that we are on the earth through the strength of the sun.

5. Plank. Exhale. Bring both legs back behind you and balance in Plank. Push out at your heels for strength. This represents finding a balance between the sun and the earth. Pause.

6. Snake pose. This is a transitional pose that Joan calls the Snake pose, where you sort of "snake" into the next pose. Exhale further. Bring your knees, chest, and chin to the floor. Keep your tailbone up off the ground. You are thanking the earth.

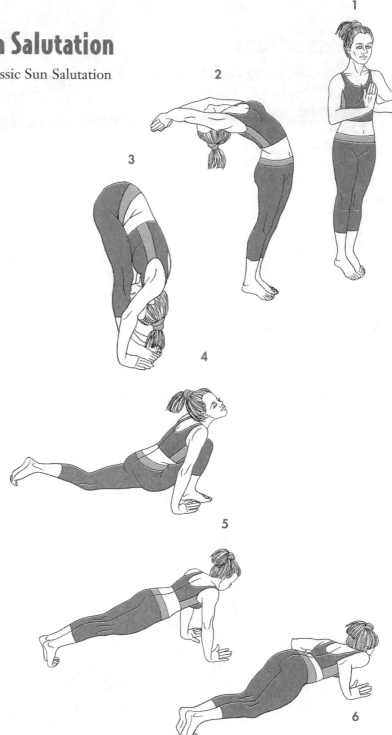

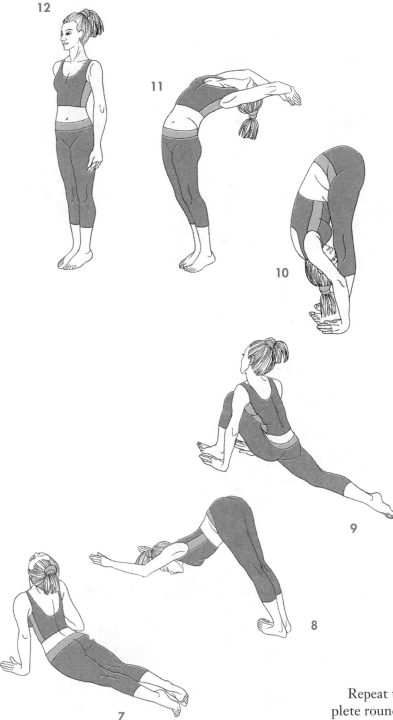

7. Upward Facing Dog. Inhale into Upward Facing Dog and look up. Let the sun's warmth strengthen you.

8. Downward Facing Dog. Exhale and push up into Downward Facing Dog pose, lengthening your spine. Let the strength of the sun enter your spine.

9. Lunge. Inhale as you bring your left foot forward. Look up and thank the sun as you proceed on your journey.

10. Standing Forward Bend. Exhale and bring both legs together. With your palms alongside your feet, humbly devote yourself to the sun. Open yourself to the sun's kind and steady energy.

11. Arms Extended. Inhale as you bring your arms and body up, tilting into a slight backbend, again embracing the sun with love.

12. Mountain pose. Exhale as you bring your hands back into the prayer position, standing in tadasana, Mountain pose.

Repeat the entire sequence again for a complete round. For the second half-round, bring your right leg back first to create a balance.

Easing into the Pose: Seated Sun Salutations

For some people, Sun Salutation is simply too difficult, strenuous, or not physically possible. If this sounds like you, try seated Sun Salutation, a gentler and less-strenuous version but a vinyasana nevertheless. Use the following figures for this Sun Salutation adaptation. Don't forget to move through this vinyasana twice so you have a chance to use both legs. All the yoga postures can be adapted for use with chairs. Place a stool, preferably with a hard seat (not upholstered) a few inches from a wall, or use a straight, hard-backed chair. It just takes some creativity and knowledge on the part of your teacher.

1. **Namaste.** Sit comfortably on a firm, straight-backed chair or a stool placed a few inches from a wall with your feet planted on the ground, your palms together in front of your chest in prayer position (namaste).

2. **Arms Extended.** Inhale and raise your arms straight up, stretching your shoulders, arms, and upper back.

3. **Seated Forward Bend.** Exhale and drop your hands toward the floor, folding your body over your thighs. Relax and breathe for a moment.

4. **Knee to Chest.** Inhale and return to an upright seated position as you raise your right knee off the ground and hold it gently with your hands, tipping your head back just slightly.

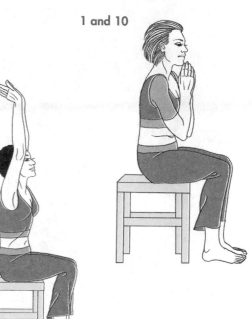

1 and 10

2

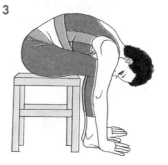

3

4

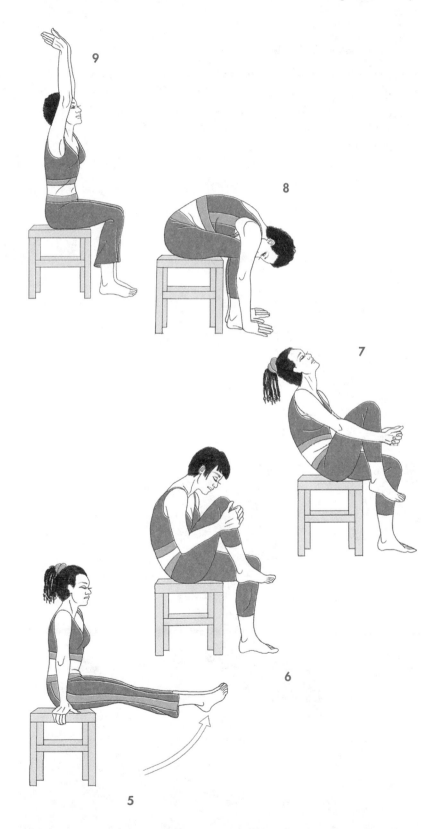

5. Leg Extension. Exhale and extend your legs forward as you grasp the sides of the chair with your hands. Depending on the stability of your chair, you may want to lift one leg at a time instead.

6. Knee to Chest, Head Down. Inhale and lower yourself back to the chair, then exhale and bend your extended leg, bringing your knee into your chest again, but this time keeping your head tilted forward toward your knee.

7. Knee to Chest, Head Up. Inhale and continue to hold your bent knee, but lean your head back slowly and looking up.

8. Seated Forward Bend. Exhale and gently lower your leg to the floor, bringing your entire body back down over your thighs and dropping your hands to the floor beside your feet.

9. Arms Extended. Inhale and raise your torso up again as you extend your arms overhead.

10. Namaste. Exhale and return your hands to prayer position in front of your chest. Then repeat the Sun Salutation with the opposite leg.

Chandra Namaskara: Moon Salutation

This Moon Salutation vinyasana restores vitality, strength, and flexibility to the entire body. It also improves digestion through the continual compression of the intestinal tract. *Chandra* means "moon," and just as the Sun Salutation greets and honors the sun, so Chandra Namaskara (*SHAHN-drah nah-MAHS-kah-rah*) greets and honors the moon. Try practicing this vinyasana outside on a clear evening when the moon is in full view. Serenity!

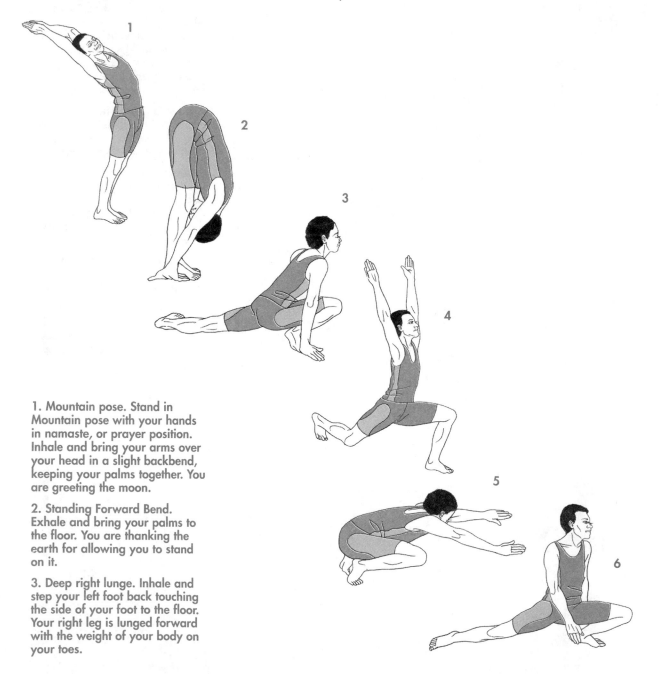

1. Mountain pose. Stand in Mountain pose with your hands in namaste, or prayer position. Inhale and bring your arms over your head in a slight backbend, keeping your palms together. You are greeting the moon.

2. Standing Forward Bend. Exhale and bring your palms to the floor. You are thanking the earth for allowing you to stand on it.

3. Deep right lunge. Inhale and step your left foot back touching the side of your foot to the floor. Your right leg is lunged forward with the weight of your body on your toes.

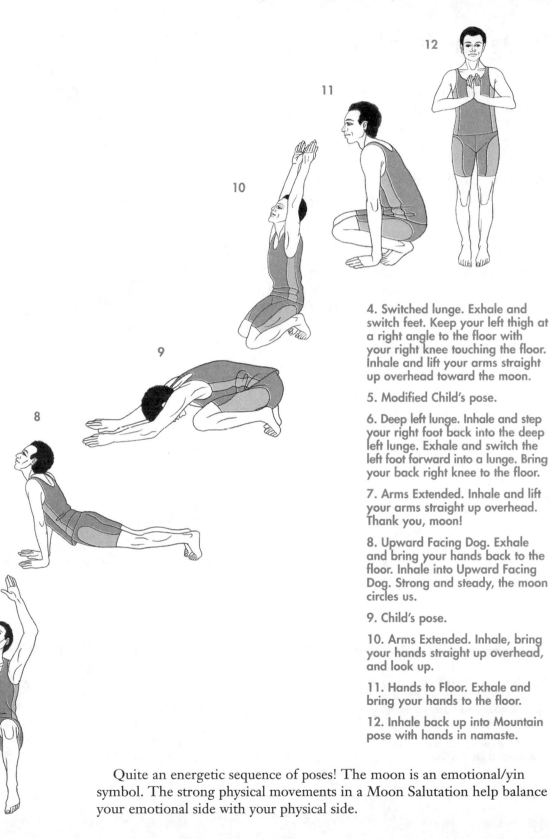

4. **Switched lunge.** Exhale and switch feet. Keep your left thigh at a right angle to the floor with your right knee touching the floor. Inhale and lift your arms straight up overhead toward the moon.

5. **Modified Child's pose.**

6. **Deep left lunge.** Inhale and step your right foot back into the deep left lunge. Exhale and switch the left foot forward into a lunge. Bring your back right knee to the floor.

7. **Arms Extended.** Inhale and lift your arms straight up overhead. Thank you, moon!

8. **Upward Facing Dog.** Exhale and bring your hands back to the floor. Inhale into Upward Facing Dog. Strong and steady, the moon circles us.

9. **Child's pose.**

10. **Arms Extended.** Inhale, bring your hands straight up overhead, and look up.

11. **Hands to Floor.** Exhale and bring your hands to the floor.

12. Inhale back up into Mountain pose with hands in namaste.

Quite an energetic sequence of poses! The moon is an emotional/yin symbol. The strong physical movements in a Moon Salutation help balance your emotional side with your physical side.

Create Your Own Flow

The Sun and Moon Salutations are popular vinyasanas because they combine a series of poses that so nicely balance each other (a back-bend, then a forward bend, and so on). But you, too, can create your own series of poses. Just keep them balanced—forward with backward, exhale with inhale, upright with inverted, one side with the other side, an expansion with a contraction, and so on. This will become easier as you familiarize yourself with the poses in this book.

Here are a few suggestions to get you started. All poses mentioned here are described elsewhere in this book or are explained here.

Warm Wonder Vinyasana

This vinyasana is quick, invigorating, and incredibly warming. We love to do this on a chilly winter evening before bed, or to warm up in the morning on a crisp fall day.

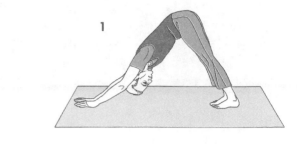

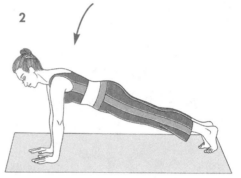

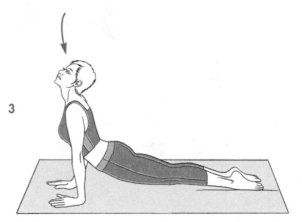

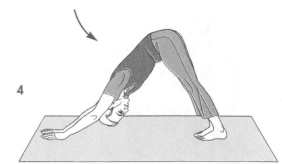

1. Downward Facing Dog.

2. Inhale and flow into Plank.

3. Exhale, bend your elbows, and lower your body straight to the floor. Inhale and push yourself up into Upward Facing Dog.

4. Exhale and push back into Downward Facing Dog.

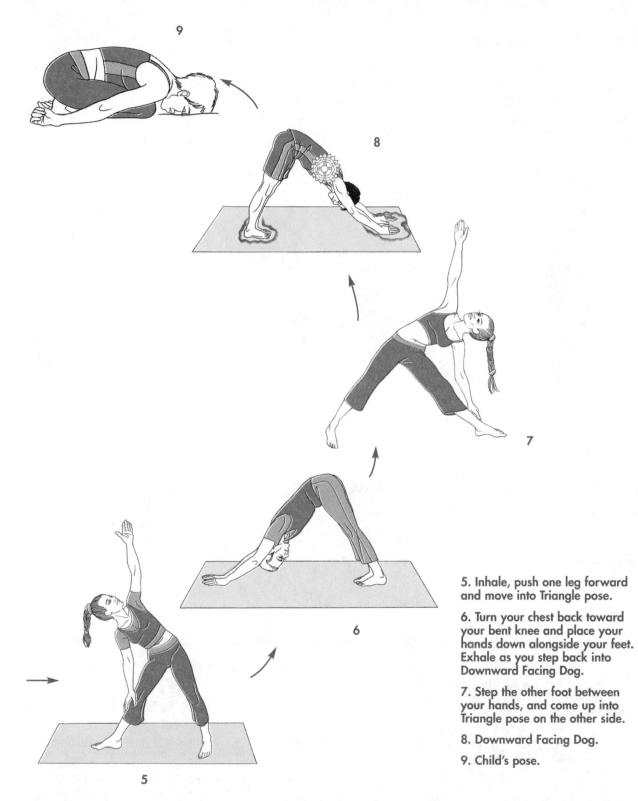

5. Inhale, push one leg forward and move into Triangle pose.

6. Turn your chest back toward your bent knee and place your hands down alongside your feet. Exhale as you step back into Downward Facing Dog.

7. Step the other foot between your hands, and come up into Triangle pose on the other side.

8. Downward Facing Dog.

9. Child's pose.

Solar Flare Vinyasana

This is a super-powered vinyasana that strengthens the body as it brings strength, confidence, and a feeling of self-possession to the bodymind. It's great before you have to give a speech or go on a first date or otherwise radiate confidence!

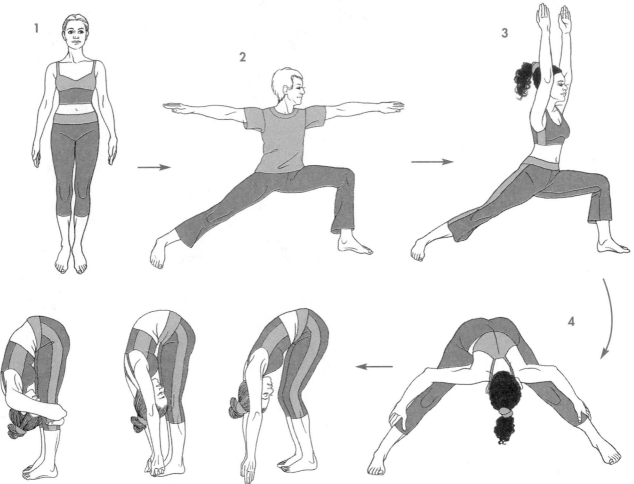

1. Mountain pose.

2. Warrior 2. Jump your feet three to four feet apart and assume Warrior 2.

3. Warrior 1. Hold for a few breaths, then turn to face forward with your arms overhead in Warrior 1. Hold for a few breaths. Switch to the other side, doing Warrior 1 and 2 in the other direction.

4. Legs Wide Forward Bend. Now, keeping your feet separated, turn your entire body to face forward and bend straight over with your knees straight. Bring your hands toward the floor and hold for a few breaths.

5. Standing Forward Bend. Come back up, jump your feet together, bend your knees, reach down through your fingertips for your toes. Slowly straighten your legs to further stretch the hamstrings. Breathe deeply. Rest.

Mild and Mindful Vinyasana

This is a calming and meditative vinyasana that helps you focus your mind as you relax your body.

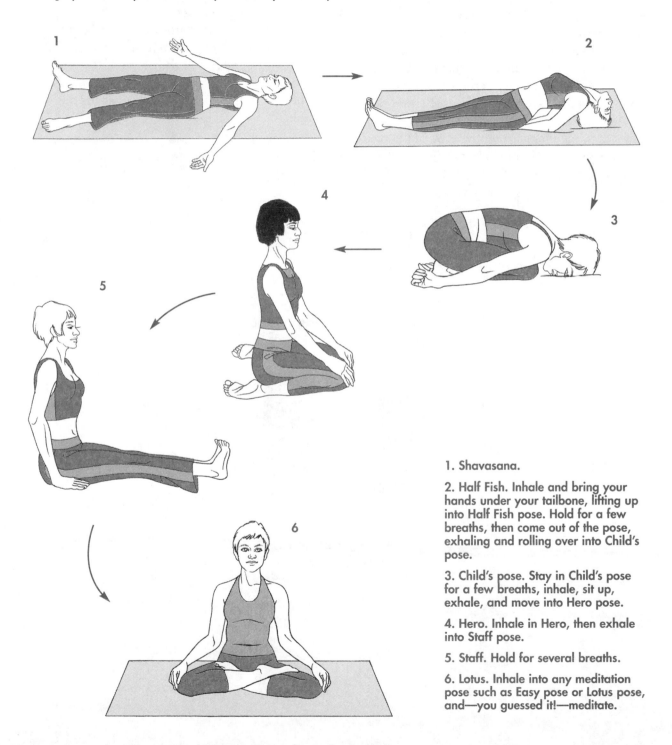

1. Shavasana.

2. Half Fish. Inhale and bring your hands under your tailbone, lifting up into Half Fish pose. Hold for a few breaths, then come out of the pose, exhaling and rolling over into Child's pose.

3. Child's pose. Stay in Child's pose for a few breaths, inhale, sit up, exhale, and move into Hero pose.

4. Hero. Inhale in Hero, then exhale into Staff pose.

5. Staff. Hold for several breaths.

6. Lotus. Inhale into any meditation pose such as Easy pose or Lotus pose, and—you guessed it!—meditate.

Moving with the Universe

While many yoga poses imitate animals or structures in nature (mountains, trees, and so on), a vinyasana imitates the rhythm and movement of the natural world. The human body is like a microcosm of the universe, with its own internal rhythms and movements. At the atomic level, the very atoms that make up everything are like tiny universes. Beyond our bodies, the world is full of cycles: the seasons, the years, the moons spinning around the planets, the planets spinning around the sun, the entire galaxy revolving.

A vinyasana helps us feel like a part of this magnificent, intricate cycle. As the sun, moon, and earth all move in concert, so our bodies move in concert through a vinyasana. Everything is moving to a sacred rhythm, ancient and eternal, and the rhythm wouldn't be the same if any one thing did not move with it. We are all part of a wave in the ocean of the universe. When we move, we are doing what comes naturally, what makes us a part of the whole.

Now if that's not a good reason to do a vinyasana every day, we don't know what is!

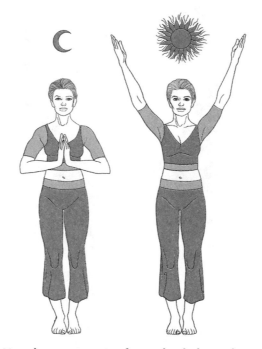

Yoga honors opposing forces that balance the human body within the powerful yet delicate balances of the universal body.

Ouch!

When performing Sun Salutation, keep your awareness focused. If you go too fast, your devotional frame of mind may sway. Go fast enough to keep the movements flowing and get your body warm, but not so fast that you don't feel in control of your movements or breath.

The Least You Need to Know

◆ A vinyasana, such as the Sun or Moon Salutation, is a sequence of postures strung together and performed in a series of flowing movements.

◆ A vinyasana is coordinated with the breath and the mind so that body, breath, and mind are integrated.

◆ The Sun Salutation is the most well-known vinyasana, but many others exist, and you can even create your own by creating sequences of poses that balance each other.

◆ Vinyasanas are great exercise for body and soul.

In This Chapter

◆ Why a little yoga goes a long way

◆ Quick five-minute yoga

◆ Calm, collected 15-minute yoga

◆ Inversions: a new perspective on life

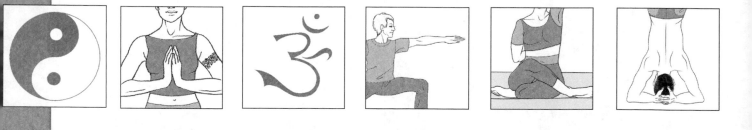

Chapter 17

Yoga in Five Minutes or Fifteen Minutes

Will five minutes of yoga really do you any good? You bet your hurried self it will! Some yoga poses can make a big difference when you are stressed or need a quick energy boost. Try peppering these five-minute yoga sessions throughout your day to bring you serenity and balance.

For more detailed instructions on how to do any of these poses, see their original descriptions from previous chapters. Each pose is listed in the table of contents and the index for easy reference.

Yoga in Five Minutes

Here are three quick yoga sessions to use whenever you have a spare five minutes—and who doesn't have five spare minutes at least once a day?

Session 1: Butterfly Take Flight

Let this movement help keep your seated meditation practice a wakeful one. Hold each pose for three breaths, then move into the next pose. Go back and forth and feel your energy soar, then return to your meditative pose. Repeat if you begin to feel sleepy again.

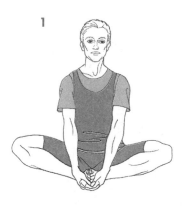

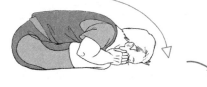

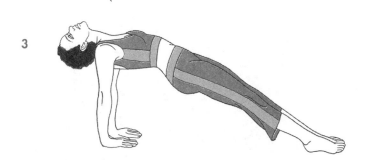

1. **Butterfly.** Relax into Butterfly pose, bringing your heels in toward your body only as far as you can still keep your spine straight, and bow forward. Hold for several breaths.

2. **Staff.** Straighten your legs and bring your hands to the floor directly under your shoulders, keeping your arms straight and fingers pointing forward. Hold Staff pose for several breaths.

3. **Upward Facing Plank.** Flow into Upward Facing Plank pose, holding for several breaths with strong arms and a straight body.

Session 2: Triple Stretch

Feel the full stretch of bodymindspirit in the powerful relationships inherent in this strength-producing sequence. Move slowly from one pose to the other, then repeat on the other side. Don't forget to breathe fully throughout this sequence.

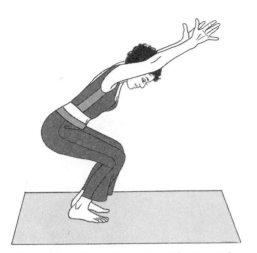

1. Lightning Bolt. Move into Lightning Bolt pose, breathing deeply, and arms straight up over your head, palms facing inward.

2. Warrior 1. Continue to ground yourself with your legs as you move into Warrior 1, lifting with your torso.

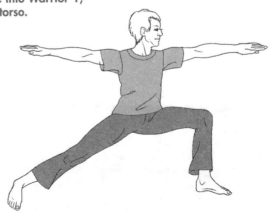

3. Warrior 2. Bring the arms down parallel with the shoulders, Warrior 2. Breathe in strength and confidence. Exhale as you change sides.

Lengthen and Balance

These poses balance, lengthen, and strengthen the body for an infusion of serenity, grace, and confidence. When you've completed this sequence, repeat, and ending in Prayer pose.

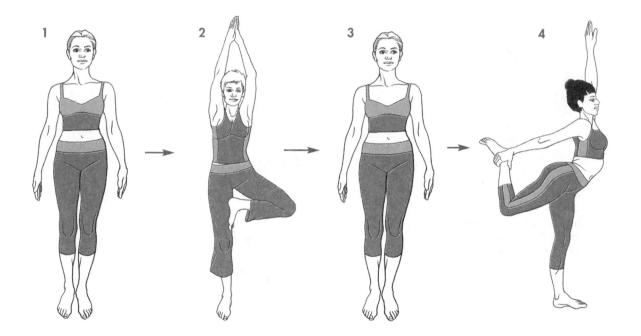

1. Mountain pose.

2. Tree. Move into Tree pose, balancing first on one side and then on the other.

3. Mountain pose. Come back to Mountain and rest for several breaths as you feel your body re-centering.

4. Shiva, or Dancer pose. Move into Dancer pose, opening the chest and fully expanding the front of your body. Repeat with the other leg.

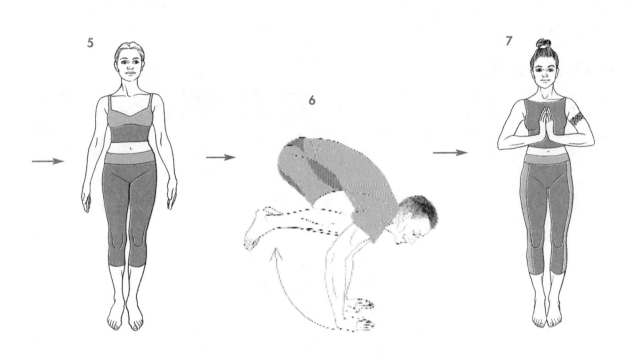

5. **Mountain pose.** Again, return to Mountain pose, feeling your body re-centering as you breathe.

6. **Crow.** Squat down into Crow pose and feel the front of your body contracting for balance.

7. **Prayer pose.** End in Prayer pose, to give thanks: namaste!

Yoga in Fifteen Minutes

When you've got a little more time but still not a lot, try any of these three 15-minute yoga sessions. The first will help relax and center you. The second will energize your bodymind and help you gain perspective. The third will pump you up!

Session 1: Calm and Collected

This 15-minute sequence is perfect for relaxing after a long and stressful day or when you've been going too fast for too long and just need to put on the brakes for a precious quarter of an hour.

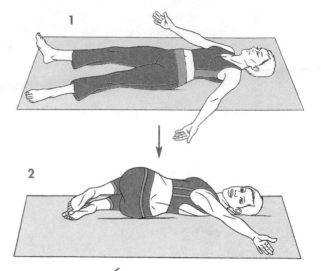

1. Relaxation. Spend a few minutes in shavasana of total relaxation, releasing your thoughts and physical tensions.

2. Lying Down Spinal Twist. Loosen your spine by drawing your knees straight up and twisting slowly, first one way, then the other. Hold and relax into each side for at least several breaths

3. Seated Spinal Twist. Further lengthen and twist your spine in Seated Spinal Twist, slowly rotating from one side, taking a few breaths there, and then from the other side. Breathe deeply.

4. Cow. Open your shoulders, expand your chest, and open your hips by doing Cow pose in a cross-legged position.

5. Scales. Release your arms to the floor and use your strength to raise your body and crossed legs in Scales pose.

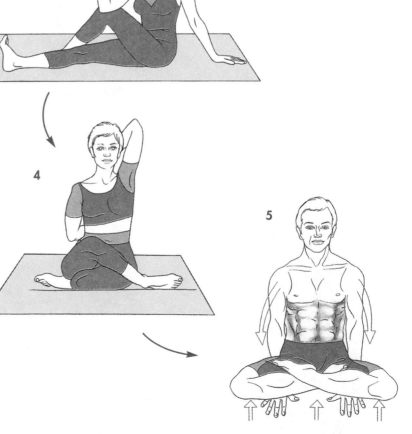

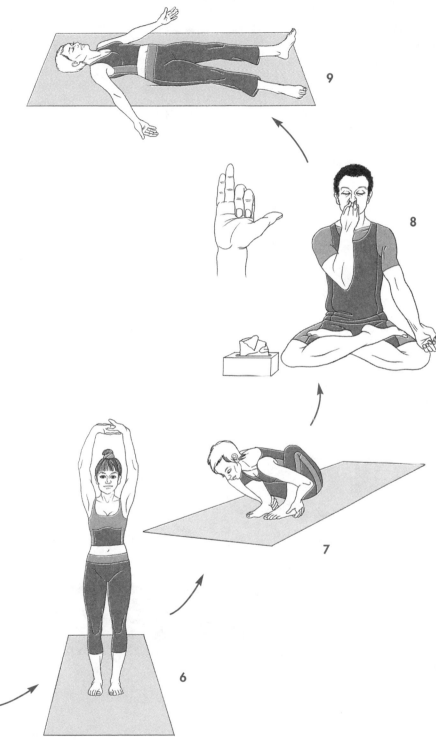

6. Mountain. Come to standing and stretch your body out with several deep breaths in Mountain pose. Bring your arms overhead to extend the stretch further.

7. Crouching pose. Squat down into Crouching pose and hold your ankles. Breathe!

8. Alternate Nostril Breathing in Lotus or Easy pose. Crossing your legs into a seated meditative pose such as Easy pose or Lotus pose, center yourself through the calming effects of the pranayama technique called Alternate Nostril Breathing to bring the emotional and physical aspects of your body into balance.

9. Shavasana. Return to shavasana to rest, release, and renew once more.

Session 2: Inversion Interest

Take a load off your feet and give yourself a whole new perspective with this 15-minute inversion sequence.

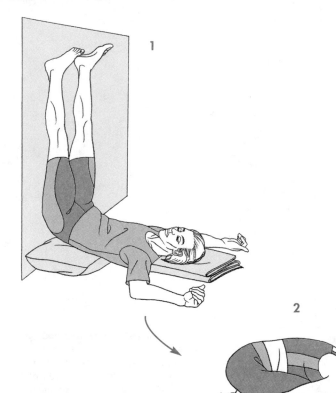

1

2

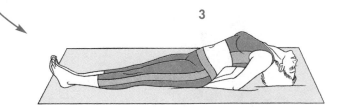

3

1. Wallflower Stretch. Begin by resting in this position for a few minutes with your legs and feet supported by a wall.

2. Child's pose. Slowly push yourself away from the wall, roll over, and come into Child's pose to balance the stretch of the hamstrings with a gentle contraction of the hamstrings.

3. Half Fish. Roll over again and stretch into Half Fish pose, opening your chest, expanding your heart and stretching your legs.

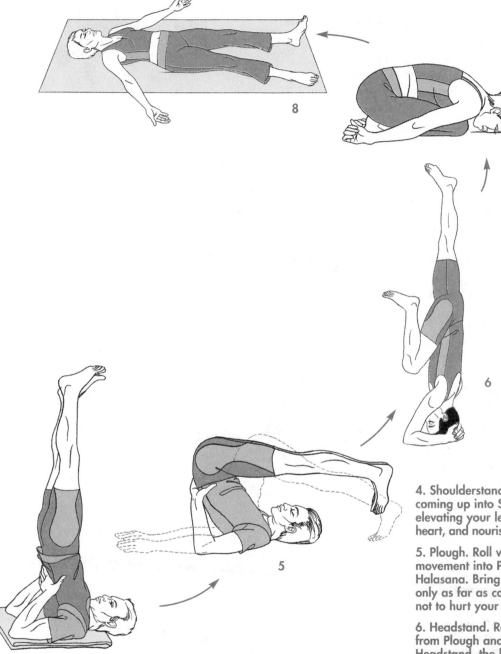

4. Shoulderstand. Balance Fish by coming up into Shoulderstand, elevating your legs, relaxing your heart, and nourishing your thyroid.

5. Plough. Roll with a controlled movement into Plough pose or Halasana. Bring your feet back only as far as comfortable so as not to hurt your spine.

6. Headstand. Roll back down from Plough and move into Headstand, the king of all poses. Spend some time there. Your mind and heart deserve it!

7. Child's pose. Relax back into Child's pose.

8. Shavasana. Finally, end with a full relaxation in shavasana.

Session 3: Move and Groove

Let this 15-minute session rock your world! It's great for getting geared up before you need to approach a task or project with lots of positive energy, whether it's an office party, a speech in front of your class, or dinner with the in-laws.

1 and 11

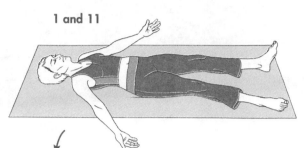

1. Shavasana. Prepare for this energizing sequence by releasing tensions to approach your practice of vinyasana calmly.

2. Pranayama Single Leg Lifts. Breath guides you as you inhale …

3. … switch to Double Leg Lifts, inhale up and exhale down; do what you can with comfort.

4. Knees to Chest. Bend your knees and hold each knee to your chest for several breaths to relax your back.

5. Half Bridge. Expand the front part of your body and open your shoulders by lifting your body up into Half Bridge pose.

6. Downward Facing Dog. Lower from Bridge, roll over, and go into Downward Facing Dog.

7. Handstand. Lift your body up into Handstand. Give your arms a workout in this strength-building balance pose, extending your spine and balancing Bridge pose.

8. Child's pose. Relax and be nurtured, resting in the universal womb of Child's pose.

9. Modified Pigeon. Come back up and stretch one leg straight back to open your hips and balance the stretches of this sequence.

10. Kneeling. In a final reflection, sit and hold your knees. Breathe slowly and deeply.

11. Shavasana. Ahhhh … relax, release ….

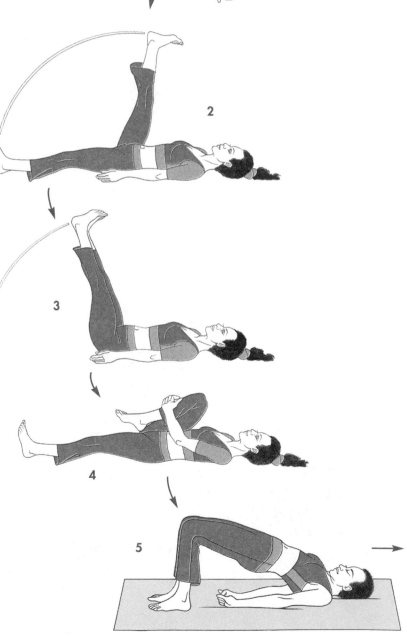

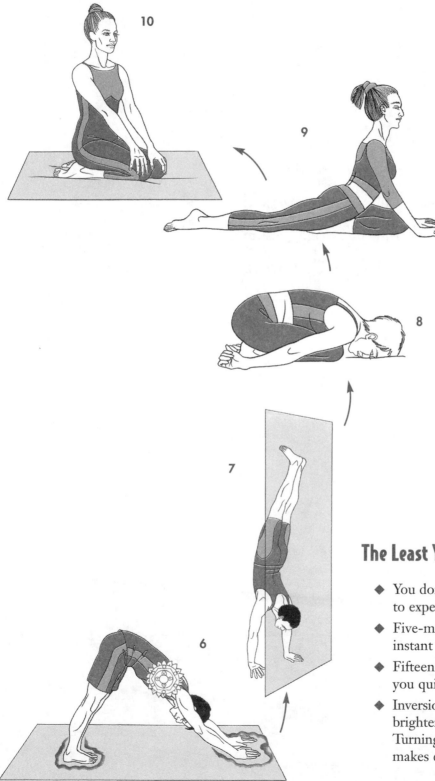

The Least You Need to Know

◆ You don't have to have a lot of time to experience a lot of yoga.

◆ Five-minute yoga sessions bring you instant calm or a burst of energy.

◆ Fifteen-minute yoga sessions help you quickly regain calmness.

◆ Inversions in a 15-minute session brighten your normal outlook. Turning your world upside down makes everything feel right side up!

In This Chapter

- ◆ Total yoga relaxation mode
- ◆ A sample 30-minute yoga session
- ◆ A sample 60-minute yoga session
- ◆ Daily sessions help you get bodymindspirit in balance

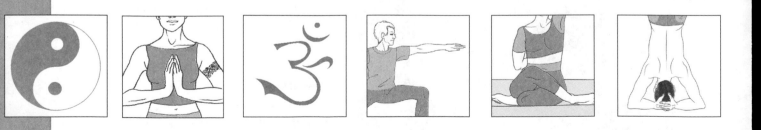

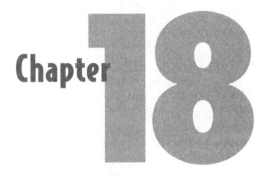

Chapter 18

Yoga in Thirty Minutes or an Hour

Sometimes it's nice to stop hurrying and spend a more dedicated chunk of time on yoga at least once or twice a week. You might enjoy it so much that you'll decide that a daily 30 minutes or an hour are just what you need. These sessions give you time to really sink into your yoga, spend as much time as you need to spend in each pose, and feel supremely and luxuriously *not* rushed.

Thirty-Minute Session: The All-Over

We think a 30-minute daily yoga session is the perfect foundation to combine with an hourly yoga class once or twice a week. This amount of time spent in daily practice helps you to maintain your practice and your yoga bodymind balance all week long.

Following is a sample 30-minute session we've put together. As you become more familiar with yoga poses, you can create your own 30-minute sessions. You can also ask your yoga teacher for options.

The following is a great all-over balancing series of vigorous yoga postures. It's both relaxing and really feels like exercise (because, of course, it *is* exercise!). We love to do this sequence to wake up in the morning or to counter that late-afternoon sag time.

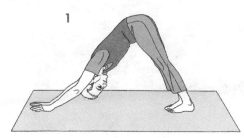

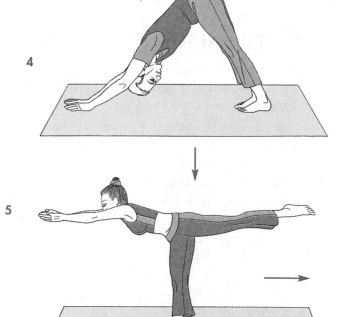

1. Downward Facing Dog. Begin your session with Downward Facing Dog, a great strength-building, spine-lengthening, overall-good-for-beginning stretch.

2. Lunge. As you exhale, step one leg forward into a Lunge and hold for several breaths.

3. Triangle. Expand Lunge by twisting to one side and straightening up into Triangle pose.

4. Downward Facing Dog. Relax back into Downward Facing Dog, evening the stretch of the spine. Move into Lunge, switching legs. Repeat steps two through four.

5. Warrior 3. This time, come out of Downward Facing Dog by lunging one foot forward and straightening up into Warrior 3. Hold for several long, deep, expansive breaths.

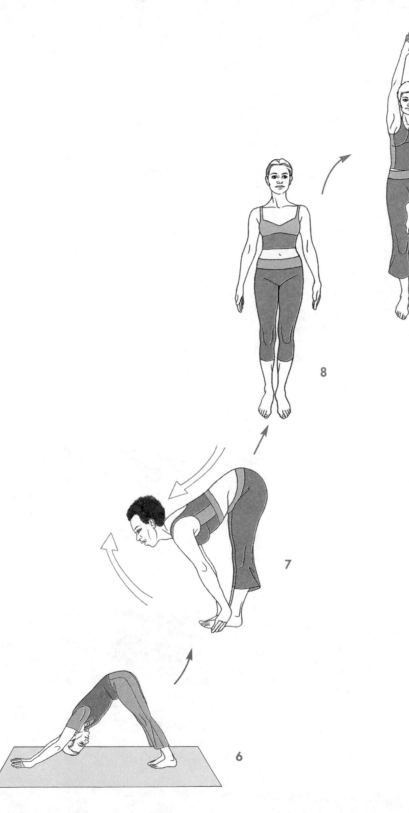

6. Downward Facing Dog. Relax back into the ever-wonderful Downward Facing Dog, then repeat the Warrior 3 on the other leg. Come back to Downward Facing Dog, jump both feet up between your hands on the floor.

7. Standing Forward Bend. Step up to the front of your mat, feet together. Straighten your torso up into Standing Forward Bend, keeping your head lifted and looking up. Feel the long stretch in your spine and breathe deeply.

8. Mountain pose. Rise up into Mountain pose and hold, firmly rooted, for a few breaths.

9. Tree. Lift one leg and both arms up to balance in Tree pose, remaining rooted but growing and breathing.

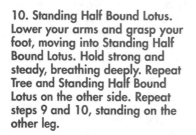

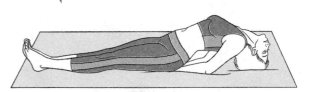

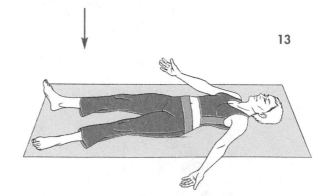

10. Standing Half Bound Lotus. Lower your arms and grasp your foot, moving into Standing Half Bound Lotus. Hold strong and steady, breathing deeply. Repeat Tree and Standing Half Bound Lotus on the other side. Repeat steps 9 and 10, standing on the other leg.

11. Extended Lightning Bolt. Sink into Extended Lightning Bolt, radiating energy into all your limbs.

12. Half Fish. Lie down on the ground, lifting your chest into Half Fish pose. Let the warmth gathered in Lightning Bolt expand further into the heart opening aspects of Fish pose.

13. Shavasana. Let the warmth of your open heart surround your body in relaxation.

Yoga in an Hour: Strength-Building Oasis of Peace

This extended yoga session is similar to what you might encounter in an hour-long yoga class. It builds strength as it builds inner peace. Take your time between poses. Spend as much time as you need to spend in each pose and enjoy the lotus flower opening inside you.

1. Namaste Breath. Choose a sitting position such as Easy pose or Lotus pose, whatever is comfortable for you, and work with slow deep breaths, raising and lowering your arms in namaste mudra, further opening your chest.

2. Rock your lower legs. Open the lower part of your body by rocking your lower legs, one at a time, rockin' and rollin' those hips.

3. Expanded spinal twist. Open your spine through this Expanded Spinal Twist, twisting on both sides.

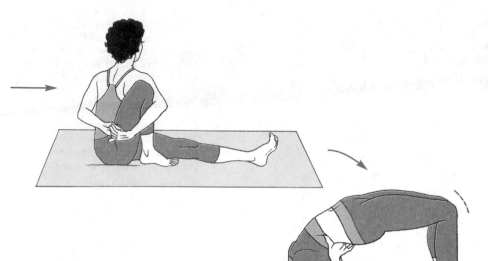

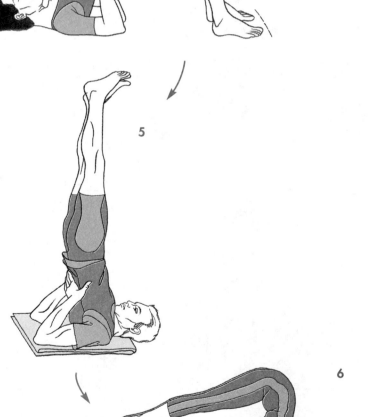

4. Bridge. Relax back and let your inhale guide you into Bridge pose. Breathe deeply.

5. Shoulderstand. Lifting one leg up at a time into shoulderstand to further the inversion. Lengthen long up to the sky.

6. Plough. Lower back to the floor and bend your knees and roll your legs over your head, lengthening and stretching your spine fully into Plough pose. Extend your arms to touch your feet. Breathe, hold for at least several breaths, then roll back up onto your heels.

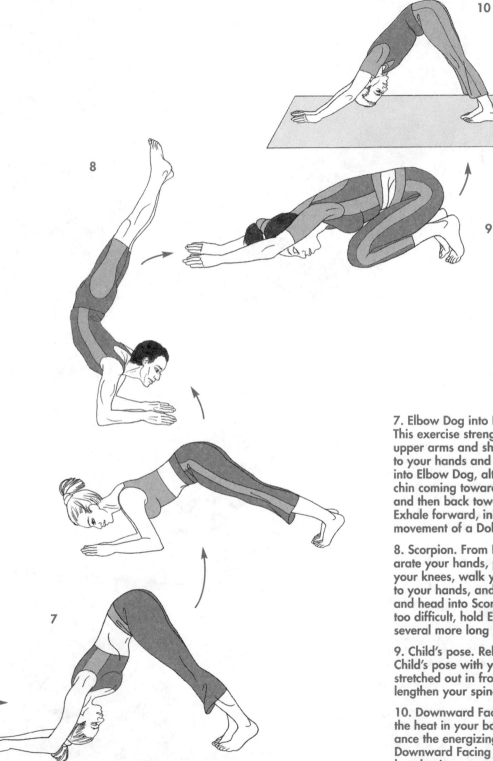

7. Elbow Dog into Dolphin pose. This exercise strengthens your upper arms and shoulders. Roll up to your hands and knees and then into Elbow Dog, alternate your chin coming toward your hands and then back toward your feet. Exhale forward, inhale back in the movement of a Dolphin.

8. Scorpion. From Elbow Dog, separate your hands, palms flat, bend your knees, walk your legs in close to your hands, and lift your torso and head into Scorpion. If this is too difficult, hold Elbow Dog for several more long breaths instead.

9. Child's pose. Relax back into Child's pose with your arms stretched out in front of you to lengthen your spine.

10. Downward Facing Dog. Feel the heat in your body as you balance the energizing effects of Downward Facing Dog by further lengthening your spine.

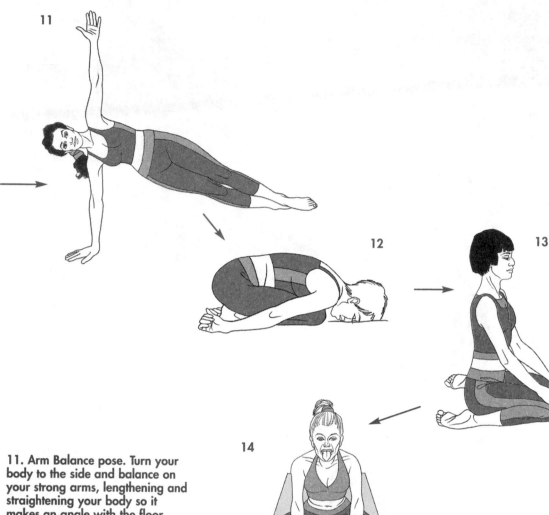

11. Arm Balance pose. Turn your body to the side and balance on your strong arms, lengthening and straightening your body so it makes an angle with the floor. Repeat on the opposite side, coming into Downward Facing Dog in between sides.

12. Child's pose. Come back down again into Child's pose, this time with your arms alongside your body. Relax.

13. Hero pose. Sit up into Hero pose. If your tailbone can touch the ground, try relaxing back into it for a fuller quadriceps stretch.

14. Lion's pose. Come back up into a release of your body in Lion's pose, either in Lotus or remaining on your knees in Hero, and roar.

15. Easy pose. Purrr. Relax and breathe in seated meditation.

These sessions should get you started. As you try yoga, you'll find you love it more and more. Poses will become easier, and you'll notice greater balance, flexibility, and strength. You'll also notice a clearer mind and a more open heart. Namaste and bliss as you join us on the yoga path; we honor your inner light!

The Least You Need to Know

◆ A daily 30- or 60-minute yoga session will keep you centered and your mindbodyspirit in balance.

◆ A 30-minute yoga session is a good way to support a weekly hour-long yoga class.

◆ Have to miss yoga class this week? Do one or two hour-long sessions for an almost-as-good-as-class bodymind workout.

◆ Make these workouts part of your routine, and you'll soon find you're enjoying the benefits of a clear mind, an open heart, and one reliable, vibrantly healthy body.

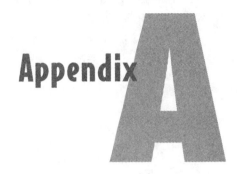

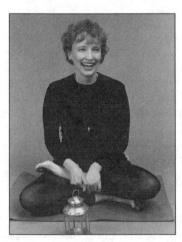

Yo Joan!

The Yo Joan column has been running on the yoyoga.com website since 1996 and has appeared biweekly in Liberty Suburban Chicago Newspapers since 1999. If you have a question for Joan, do not hesitate to write her. She does lots of yoga and gets regular massages to keep up with all her mail (and is always looking for more reasons to do more yoga and get more massages). You can write Joan at yojoan@yoyoga.com.

Yo Joan,

First of all, I would like to thank you and Eve Adamson for your book, The Complete Idiot's Guide to Yoga. *I bought it after Christmas and love it! Initially I bought it for some breathing/calming exercises that would help me as a mother of two small children; however, as well as this, it's helped me in many ways, and I find I miss yoga horribly when I don't have time or a chance to do it, even if it's only one day!*

I am wondering if you could give me some general guidelines in creating my own series of poses to do?

Dear friend,

Thanks! We've very much enjoyed putting this new edition together, too, and have added a co-author in the process. Welcome aboard, Carolyn Flynn! Now, regarding your question, keep in mind balance (hatha). If you do a forward bend, balance with a backward bend. If you twist to one side, twist to the other side. Every day try at least one pose from each of these following categories:

> Forward Bend
>
> Backward Bend
>
> Twist
>
> Balance
>
> Inversion

Occasionally close your eyes while holding the pose. Notice what your body is saying to you. This is an internal study. As your practice continues to develop, your internal awareness becomes ever more subtle.

Namaste,

Joan

Yo Joan,

I'm not quite sure if I am meditating right. When I sit quietly and my mind goes blank, is that meditating?

Dear friend,

Not necessarily. Meditation is when the mind is so focused that one actually merges with the object of meditation. This is why meditation exercises are basically concentration exercises, such as focusing on the breath, or a candle, or a sound. These concentration exercises bring the mind to a focused attention. It is very easy to drift from this focus and start dreaming of something else. The yoga yamas can help here. These yamas (observances) are *non-violence, truthfulness, non-stealing, non-greed, and non-lust.* They offer a guiding framework for our thoughts. Bringing these yamas into your practice purifies the mind so that when the mind does merge with its object of meditation, it is closer to the essence of one's reality. In yoga,

this would be considered a heightened, blissful state of awareness. So, when you're feeling down, move around, but when you're feeling great, meditate.

Namaste,

Joan

Yo Joan,

Violence ruins so many lives. It's like a spreading disease for which no one knows the cure. We all think that our lives will never be touched by violence, but odds are increasing that it will happen. I heard that yoga teaches nonviolence. How?

Dear friend,

Violence is indeed a part of this world. Some would say it's an inevitable part. Yet it is important to reflect upon which came first, the violence within our fists or the violence within our minds. As the world around us continually changes, yoga sharpens our awareness of how the inner world of our thoughts and emotions shapes the outer world of our experiences. By observing where the judgmental mind travels, we can begin to guide the mind into more peaceful territory and into a less judgmental nature. In this way, we become more active instead of reactive. To begin this process, simply try releasing a negative thought or tendency through the exhale of your breath. Something so seemingly simple can really be quite difficult to do. This is why regular practice is necessary, and the support of a yoga class can be encouraging to the process.

Namaste,

Joan

Yo Joan,
Can yoga heal depression?

Dear friend,
Certainly some depressions require medical attention. Do not hesitate to seek this if your depression persists. Still, many of us are not aware of how the simple ways we hold our bodies can significantly affect our health.

Try this easy exercise:

Hunch your back and round your shoulders. Notice your emotions as you do this. Take several breaths here. Now, bring your shoulders up toward your ears and then draw them down away from your ears. Open your chest. Lengthen your spine upright. Bring your chin parallel with the ground. Take several deep breaths here. Notice your emotions now. Did you see any slight changes? Perhaps even some major ones?

If you are not in good shape or if you find discipline difficult, you may find even the simplest yoga breathing exercises of pranayama exhausting to do alone at home. A yoga class can help motivate you to stick with the important health building techniques of pranayama. And, even though yoga is non-competitive, a yoga class can challenge and encourage you along in your practice of the yoga poses as well.

Namaste,

Joan

Yo Joan,
Can yoga improve my sex life?

Dear friend,
Yes. Because self-awareness is a part of yoga practice, and the more aware you are, the more you have access to all of your emotions. Your physical bliss will be more blissful and your physical joy will be more joyful.

Namaste,

Joan

Yo Joan,
I have a question about singing, seeing you have been a singer you might understand. Are singing and yoga related in the breathing techniques that are used? I find it hard to free my voice and find I'm unable to reach high notes as a result, could it be something to do with blocked energies? Would it help my singing if I started yoga and meditation?

Dear friend,
Yoga helped me in my singing but it wasn't a matter of singing higher notes; it was a matter of finding and expressing my inner voice. The clearer the inner voice is, the clearer the outer voice becomes. Mercury Chakra is in the throat region and is the seat of our communications and expressions. So, certainly poses that can open the throat region, such as Shoulderstand and Fish pose, can be beneficial to singers. Yoga can help actualize any gift you have.

Namaste,

Joan

Yo Joan,
I "googled" kundalini and it said it is dangerous if experienced alone or without a practitioner familiar with kundalini. Also, it said the experience is out of body and uncontrollable! Would I experience this "kundalini" by practicing with my DVDs at home alone? Does this happen spontaneously without my wanting it to happen?

Dear friend,
First, take a deep breath and exhale slowly. Yoga is about decreasing stress, not increasing it. According to yogic thought, the basis of our innate energy (kundalini) is pure beautiful joy beyond description. Layers of illusions exist that often prevent us from seeing or realizing this incredible energy. The yogi's path is to remove the layers of illusions that prevent us from living the energetic reality of inner peace;

this path begins through the practice of non-violence. By bringing nonviolence into one's awareness, and gradually into one's actions, one starts to realize a shift in awareness and a purer energy. Also keep in mind, my friend, in the end, when all is said and done, a google can actually be a giggle sometimes.

Namaste,

Joan

Yo Joan,

How do you pronounce your last name? Is it Buddha–luv–ski or Booty-love-ski?

Dear friend,

I prefer Buddy–LOVE–ski, with an accent on the "love." In reality, we do not know if the Buddha loved to ski, but we do know that I am your buddy.

Namaste,

Joan

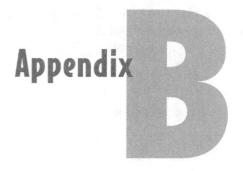

Appendix B

Meet Your Chakras

In yogic thought, the body contains energy centers called chakras (literally "wheels") that store energy, or the life force, prana. As energy moves through the body via meridians or energy channels, it collects and pools in the chakras, sort of like lakes along a network of rivers and underground streams. Westerners would interpret the chakras as nerve centers, but they are much more than this. They are centers of psychospiritual energy that don't precisely correspond to any tangible physical structure.

Although the body contains many energy centers and sub-energy centers, there are seven primary chakras along the midline of the body. Different people have different names for these chakras and place them in slightly different locations, but in essence, most agree that these seven chakras begin at the base of the spine where the kundalini energy lies coiled and waiting to be activated so it can continue along the spinal cord, ending in the seventh chakra at the crown of the head.

Different traditions associate different things with each chakra: which body parts, emotions, and thoughts each chakra governs; which colors each chakra radiates; which areas of our personality each chakra represents.

There are no pervasive Western names for the chakras; people name them after colors, mantra syllables, the elements, and so on. Yoga scholar Georg Feuerstein names chakras things like "root prop wheel," "jewel city wheel," and "wheel of the unstruck sound." None of these naming systems is arbitrary; the chakras do indeed correspond to many different energies.

This appendix introduces you to the seven chakras as we experience them. As yoga works to move our consciousness toward the center, we utilize planet names in understanding these spheres of moving energy. Through planetary symbols revolving around the sun, we are studying the universe within us—a truly universal concept. Remember that although we experience the chakras centered on certain anatomical areas, the chakras exist not only in us and but also beyond our physical bodies as wheels of energy. All chakras must be activated or awakened for full enlightenment, which is not an easy process. Awakening a chakra—releasing the energy that flows through your spine—can take years, perhaps lifetimes! Its hard work to *en*-lighten up!

The following table shows you exactly what each chakra governs.

Chakras at a Glance

Chakra	Keyword	Planet	Color	Location	Physical	Emotional
1st	Root	Saturn	Red	Base of spine	Elimination, releasing; sense of smell	Security and survival; instinctual responses; needs and drives; family
2nd	Creativity	Jupiter	Orange	Lower abdomen, below belly button, above genitals	Reproductive organs; taste; body's water content	Sexuality; passions; creativity
3rd	Power	Mars	Yellow	Abdomen, behind belly button	Digestion; consumption	Action; sense of self; personal power; integrity; self-esteem; personal code of ethics
4th	Love	Venus	Green	Heart	Cardiovascular system	Compassion; emotions toward others; transformation (love changes everything); forgiveness
5th	Expression	Mercury	Blue	Throat	Throat; tonsils; voicebox	Communication skills; your choices; your affirmations
6th	Truth	Sun	Indigo	Middle of forehead	Mental processes	Clear perception; knowledge; recognition of truth
7th	Inspiration	Thousand-Petalled Lotus	Violet	Crown	Integration of whole self; body, mind, and spirit	Spiritual enlightenment; unity

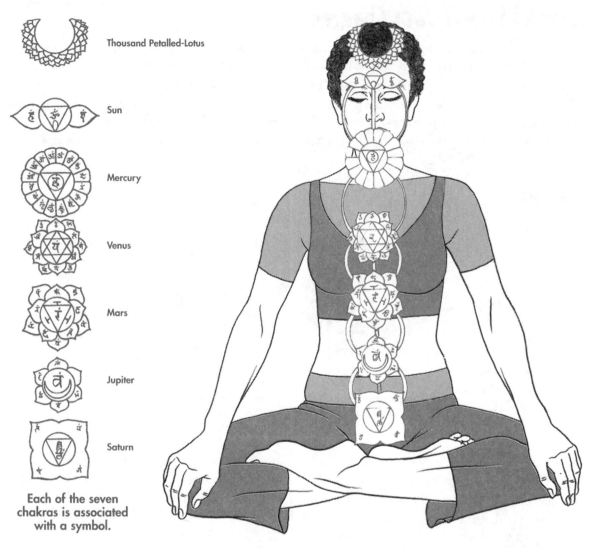

Thousand Petalled-Lotus

Sun

Mercury

Venus

Mars

Jupiter

Saturn

Each of the seven chakras is associated with a symbol.

The seven chakras are distinctive energy centers, often depicted as different lotus-petalled shapes drawn along the human spine. Doing Hatha Yoga activates the chakras.

Poses to Power Your Chakras

Certain yoga poses can make releasing and opening the chakras easier. We'll show you a few poses for opening your chakras, which floods them with prana, energizes them, and helps balance your entire bodymind. Add a few chakra-releasing poses to your yoga routine and feel the power of prana!

Knowing what chakra is linked to a problem—a blockage or an overflow of energy in your body is helpful—but how do you activate or heal a chakra? Try these chakra-opening poses, or simply focus on a chakra and its associated color during shavasana or sitting meditation, to help release, activate, and empower that chakra.

Open Pose

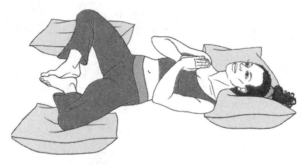

Open pose releases the chakras in the lower half of the torso. It is also excellent for relaxation and meditation.

1. Lie down on the floor on your back with a pillow under your head.

2. Bend your knees and bring the soles of your feet together, letting your knees drop to the floor. If this is uncomfortable, or if your back overarches, place a pillow under each knee.

3. Bring your palms together in front of your heart in namaste. Breathe deeply several times, focusing on releasing your lower chakras. Feel the prana flowing through them.

4. If this pose brings strong feelings or emotions to the surface, simply watch them as they drift to the surface. Then, when you're ready, simply let them go with your exhale. Keep breathing and relaxing until you feel calm, energized, and ready to move on.

Prana Arch

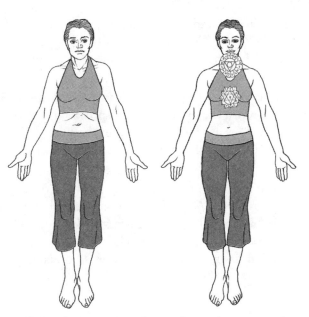

Slumped posture crowds your internal organs and impedes the flow of prana through the heart and throat chakras. Correct posture in Prana Arch pose opens the heart and throat chakras.

In this pose, the front of your body opens, releasing tension in your chest, neck, and abdomen. Breathing deeply through this pose encourages the flow of prana through the chakras. Prana Arch helps your body balance any slumping you might normally do, correcting your posture in a way that opens your chest and throat and frees energy. Good posture gives all your internal organs more room to work and makes you feel more confident, too.

1. Stand in Mountain pose with your arms hanging loosely at your sides.

2. Inhale as you look up and just slightly behind you. At the same time, lift your hands, palms facing forward, away from your body and out to the sides, as if preparing to give someone a big hug.

3. Contract your buttock muscles to support your lower back. Don't lean back farther than is comfortable. Breathe deeply several times. On the exhale, lower your arms and head, coming back into Mountain pose.

The Healing Power of Chakras

Because each chakra governs a physical and emotional area, you may direct certain yoga poses to release blocked energy in the chakra area. For instance, difficult or strained communication could indicate a blocked Mercury chakra. Indigestion or an inability to act on your feelings could point to a blocked Mars chakra.

Triangle pose can help relieve lower back pain by releasing the lower chakras and allowing prana to flow through this area. Or to warm the extremities by spreading the heat from the heart chakra to the hands and feet, try Downward Facing Dog. Sometimes the power of two is greater than the power of one. Meditate on the chakras with a partner; concentrate on connecting with and nurturing positive energy between you.

Feeling frazzled and unfocused? Try a pose that awakens your Saturn chakra, located at the base of your spine. Overemotional or unforgiving? Try a pose that balances your Venus chakra, located behind your heart. Angry or hostile? Try a pose to balance the Mars chakra, located behind your navel. Having a problem communicating? Work with your Mercury chakra, located in the throat. Each Hatha Yoga posture is designed to awaken and balance different chakras, so practicing the right poses can be the best prescription for what ails you.

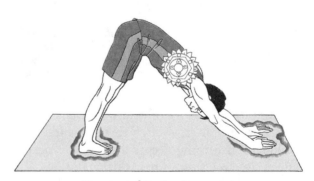

Downward Facing Dog pose.

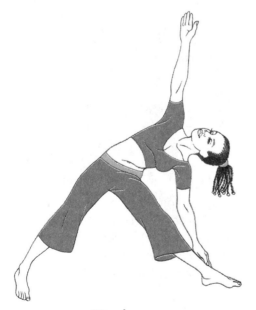

Triangle pose.

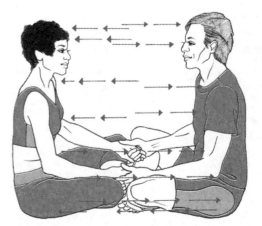

Connecting your chakras.

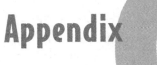

Glossary

abhinivesha   Survival instinct.

adho mukha shavasana   Downward Facing Dog; a forward bend.

adho mukha vrksasana   The Handstand; an inversion.

ahimsa   One of the yamas; nonviolence.

allopathic medicine   The traditional medicine of Western culture, which focuses on a specific disease or problem and treats it.

ananda-maya-kosha   The bliss sheath and fifth sheath of existence.

anna-maya-kosha   The physical body and first sheath of existence.

apana   A type of prana; the vital energy of excretion that flows downward and out of the body, ridding it of impurities.

aparigraha   One of the yamas; nongreed.

ardha baddha padma pashchimottanasana   Bound Half Lotus pose; a seated forward-bending pose.

ardha baddha padmottanasana   Standing Half Bound Lotus pose; an advanced balancing pose.

asanas   The postures, or exercises, of yoga designed to help you master control of your body.

Ashtanga Yoga   Literally refers to the Eight Limbs of Yoga; in Western culture, this type of yoga has come to mean a Hatha Yoga practice that includes an intense vinyasana workout.

asmita   Ego or individuality.

asteya   One of the yamas; nonstealing.

astral body   The vehicle of the spirit, corresponding with the mind; higher than the physical body, but below the causal body.

aum   A sacred sound (also referred to as om) commonly used as a mantra during meditation and representative of the absolute or oneness of the universe; a rough approximation of the sound of the universe's vibration.

avidya   Incorrect comprehension.

baddha konasana   The Butterfly; a sitting posture.

baddha padmasana   The Bound Lotus; a meditative pose.

bandha   Literally "to bind" or "to lock," bandhas are muscular locks used during postures and breathing exercises to intensify the energy of prana so it can eliminate impurities from the body.

Bhagavad Gita   One of India's most beloved and famous sacred texts, this is the epic story of Arjuna, a warrior-prince who confronts moral dilemmas and is led to a better understanding of reality through the intercession of the god Krishna.

Bhakti Yoga   Sincere, heartfelt devotion to the divine is the primary focus of this type of yoga.

bhastrika   Literally "bellows," bhastrika is a breathing technique that imitates the action of a bellows.

bhramari   Also known as Bee Breath, this breathing technique imitates the sound of a bee.

bhujangasana   The Cobra; a backbend.

brahmacharya   One of the yamas; chastity or nonlust.

brahman   The absolute, or divinity itself.

buddhi   The intellect.

cakrasana   The Wheel; a backbend.

causal body   The subtlest body, it houses the spirit; higher than the physical and astral bodies.

chakras   Centers of energy that exist between the base of your spinal column and the crown of your head.

chandra namaskara   Moon salutation; a vinyasana.

circadian rhythms   The physiological rhythms people experience throughout the course of a 24-hour day.

dandasana   The Staff; a sitting posture.

dhanurasana   The Bow; a backbend.

dharana   Orienting the mind toward a single point.

dhyana   Meditation, or the process of quieting the mind to free yourself from preconceptions and illusions.

duhkha   Pain, suffering, trouble, and discomfort; a mental state during which limitations and a profound sense of dissatisfaction are perceived.

dvesha   Refusal.

estrogen   Hormones that produce sexual changes in female mammals.

fruitarian   A person who eats only raw fruits, "vegetable fruits" like tomatoes and cucumbers, nuts, and seeds, but nothing cooked or killed.

garudasana   The Eagle; a balance posture.

ghee   Clarified butter, or butter from which all solids have been removed, leaving only the oil; a traditional Indian food.

gomukhasana   The Cow; a sitting posture.

gunas   The three primary qualities existing in the universe—sattva, rajas, and tamas—can apply to the mind and to influences on the body, such as food.

guru   Literally "dispeller of darkness," a guru is a personal spiritual advisor who helps direct the yogi toward enlightenment.

halasana   The Plough; an inversion.

Hatha Yoga   A type of yoga primarily concerned with mastering control over the physical body as a path to enlightenment; Hatha Yoga combines opposing forces to achieve balance.

Hatha-Yoga-Pradipika A fourteenth-century comprehensive guide to Hatha Yoga.

holistic medicine An approach to medicine in which the patient's entire lifestyle, environment, and personality are considered in the treatment of disease.

ida A channel on the left side of the spine through which prana moves.

ishvara-pranidhana One of the niyamas; centering on the divine.

jalandhara bandha A bandha that locks the throat.

janu shirshasana Sitting One Leg; a forward bend.

japa The process of repeating a mantra over and over for the purpose of clearing the mind.

Jnana Yoga This type of yoga emphasizes questioning, meditation, and contemplation as paths to enlightenment.

kali yuga The fourth of four ages (yuga means "age"), and the age in which we are now living; the shortest of all the ages, kali yuga is more than 432,000 years long.

kapalabhati A cleansing ritual for the respiratory tract, lungs, and sinuses; also called Skull Shining.

karma The law of cause and effect, or the movement toward balanced consciousness; everything you do, say, or even think has an immediate effect on the universe that will reverberate back to you in some way.

Karma Yoga Selfless action and service to others are emphasized in this type of yoga.

Kevali Kumbhaka A pranayama technique involving retaining the breath, it helps increase breath control and lung capacity.

koshas The five sheaths of existence that comprise the body.

Krishna A popular Hindu god.

Kriya Yoga The yoga of action and participation in life.

kundalini Literally "she who is coiled," kundalini is a psychospiritual energy force in the body that is often compared to a snake lying curled at the base of the spine, waiting to be awakened. When fully awakened, it is said to actually restructure the body, allowing the yogi to control previously involuntary bodily functions.

Kundalini Yoga This esoteric and mystical form of yoga is centered around awakening and employing kundalini energy.

kurmasana The Tortoise; a forward bend.

lacto vegetarianism A form of vegetarianism in which no meat, poultry, fish, or eggs are consumed; but milk and milk products are consumed.

lacto-ovo vegetarianism A form of vegetarianism in which no meat, poultry, or fish is consumed; but eggs, milk, and milk products are consumed.

mandalas Beautiful, usually circular, geometric designs that draw your eye to the center and are used as a center of focus in meditation.

mano-maya-kosha The mind sheath and third sheath of existence.

mantra A sound or sounds that resonate in the body and evoke certain energies during meditation.

Mantra Yoga The chanting of mantras characterizes this type of yoga.

maricyasana The Half Spinal Twist; a twisting pose.

matsyasana The Fish; a backbend.

Matsyendra A Hindu sage and one of the first teachers of Hatha Yoga.

menopause The period in a woman's life, usually somewhere between her late 30s and her early 60s, when menstruation ceases.

mudhasana Child's pose; a forward bend.

mudras Hand gestures that direct the life current through the body.

mula bandha   An anal lock.

murccha kumbkhaka   A pranayama technique also known as third eye breathing, this exercise involves breathing with a focus on the third eye, or the area between and just above the eyebrows (the sixth chakra).

nadi shodhana   A breathing exercise in which nostrils are alternated for inhalation and exhalation.

nadis   Subtle vibratory passages of psycho-spiritual energy.

namaste mudra   A mudra in which the hands are placed together in prayerlike fashion to honor the inner light.

naukasana   The Full Boat; a balance pose.

niyamas   Five observances or personal disciplines, as defined by Patanjali in his Yoga Sutras; the niyamas are saucha, santosha, tapas, svadhyaya, and ishvar-pranidhana.

om   A sacred sound (also referred to as aum) commonly used as a mantra during meditation and representative of the absolute or oneness of the universe; a rough approximation of the sound of the universe's vibration.

padma shirshasana   The Lotus Headstand; an inversion.

padmasana   The Lotus pose, a meditative posture in which the legs are crossed and each foot is placed on the opposite thigh; the pose is said to resemble the perfection of the lotus flower.

parshvottanasana   The Side Angle Stretch; a standing posture.

pavana maktasana   Also called Wind Relieving pose, this standing pose brings the knee to the chest, with head extended toward the knee.

physical body   The lowest of the three bodies, the physical body is the body we see; the other bodies are the astral body and the causal body.

pingala   A channel on the right side of the spine through which prana moves.

PMS   An acronym for premenstrual syndrome.

postpartum depression   A condition experienced by at least 50 percent of new mothers; characterized by depression, anxiety, drastic mood swings, and spontaneous weeping in the week after childbirth.

prana   A form of energy in the universe that animates all physical matter, including the human body; the vital energy of respiration and the soul of the universe.

prana-maya-kosha   The vital body and second sheath of existence.

pranayama   Breathing exercises designed to help you master control of your breath.

pratyahara   Withdrawal of the senses.

premenstrual syndrome   A syndrome experienced by some women one to two weeks before the onset of menstruation; symptoms may include irritability, depression, restlessness, back pain, bloating, and swelling.

purvottanasana   The Hands to Feet pose; a variation of the Plough; an inversion.

raga   Attachment.

Raja Yoga   Also known as The Royal Path, this type of yoga emphasizes control of the intellect to attain enlightenment.

rajas   The quality of high activity and agitation; a guna.

Rig Veda   Literally "Knowledge of Praise," the Rig Veda consists of 1,028 hymns and is the oldest known reference to yoga and possibly the oldest known text in the world.

roga   Sickness.

samadhi   The state of meditation in which ego disappears and all becomes one; a state of absolute bliss.

samyama   When in a state of samyama, the yogi has investigated, concentrated on, meditated upon, and contemplated an object or subject until everything about it is known and understood.

santosha   One of the niyamas; contentment.

sarvangasana   The Shoulderstand; an inversion.

sattva   The quality of clarity and lightness; a guna.

satya   One of the yamas; truthfulness.

saucha   One of the niyamas; purity, or inner and outer cleanliness.

setu bandha sarvangasana   The Bridge; an inversion.

shat kriyas   Purification rituals.

shavasana   Also known as Corpse pose, this pose is meant to bring the body and mind into total, conscious relaxation.

shirshasana   The Headstand; an inversion.

shodhana   Yogic cleansing rituals.

sitali   A breathing technique involving rolling the tongue, then inhaling through it like a straw; a cooling technique.

sthala basti   A yoga cleansing ritual for the colon, also called ground colon cleansing, involving the churning of the abdominal muscles.

sthira   Steadiness and alertness.

sukha   Lightness and comfort.

sukhasana   Easy pose; a meditative pose.

Suchakra   Located in the middle of your brow, this energy center is also known as the third eye, or center of unclouded perception.

surya namaskara   Sun Salutation; a vinyasana.

sushumna   A hollow passageway between pingala and ida that runs through the spinal cord, and through which kundalini can travel once it is awakened.

svadhyaya   One of the niyamas; the process of inquiring into your own nature, the nature of your beliefs, and the nature of the world's spiritual journey.

svamin   A title of respect for a spiritual person who is master of her- or himself rather than others.

svasthya   Health.

swami   The Anglicized form of svamin.

Swami Vivekananda   A guru from India who addressed the Parliament of Religions in 1893, and quickly became a popular figure; he was followed by a number of other swamis who came to the United States to teach and guide Westerners along the Eastern path of yoga.

tadasana   The Mountain; a standing posture.

tamas   The quality of heaviness and inactivity; a guna.

Tantra Yoga   This type of yoga is characterized by certain rituals designed to awaken the kundalini.

tapas   One of the niyamas; self-discipline.

Thousand-Petalled Lotus chakra   Located at the crown of the skull, this energy center is the core of self-realization, perspective, unity, and enlightenment.

Transcendental Meditation   Also known as TM, this form of meditation involves the mental repetition of a mantra.

trikonasana   The Triangle or Happy pose; a standing posture.

uddiyana bandha   A bandha that locks the abdomen.

ujjayi   A breathing exercise that produces sound in the throat with the inhalation; literally, "she who is victorious."

Upanishads   Scriptures of ancient Hindu philosophy.

urdhvamukha shvanasana   The Upward Facing Dog; a backbend.

ustrasana   The Camel; a backbend.

utkatasana   The Lightning Bolt; a standing posture.

uttanasana   Standing Head to Knee; a forward bend.

uttanatavasana   Leg Lifts.

vajrasana   Kneeling pose; a meditative pose.

vashisthasana   The Arm Balance; a balance posture.

veganism   A form of vegetarianism in which no animal products of any kind are consumed.

vegetarianism   A diet in which no meat is consumed.

vidya   Correct understanding.

vijnana-maya-kosha   The intellect sheath and fourth sheath of existence.

vinyasana   A steady flow of connected yoga asanas linked with breathwork in a continuous movement; a particularly dynamic form of yoga.

virabhadrasana   The Warrior; a standing posture.

virasana   The Hero; a sitting posture.

vrikshasana   The Tree; a balance posture.

vyadhi   Disease.

yamas   Five abstinences that purify the body and mind, as defined by Patanjali in his Yoga Sutras; the yamas are ahimsa, satya, asteya, brahmacharya, and aparigraha.

yoga mudra   Symbol of yoga. A forward bend.

Yoga Sutras   The source of Patanjali's Eight-fold Path, this collection of succinct aphorisms has largely defined the modern concept of yoga.

yogi   Someone who practices yoga.

yogic   An adjective describing things that are associated with yoga.

yogini   A female yogi.

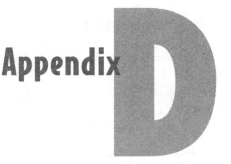

Appendix D

Along the Yoga Path: Suggested Reading

Welcome! Now that you're on your way to establishing a yoga practice with *The Complete Idiot's Guide to Yoga Illustrated, Fourth Edition,* here's how to find out more about the yoga path!

Adamson, Eve, and Linda Horning, R.D. *The Complete Idiot's Guide to Fasting.* Indianapolis: Alpha Books, 2002.

Anderson, Sandra, and Rolf Sovik, Psy.D. *Yoga: Mastering the Basics.* Honesdale, PA: The Himalayan Institute Press, 2000.

Balch, James F., and Phyllis A. Balch. *Prescription for Nutritional Healing, 2nd Edition.* Garden City Park, NY: Avery Publishing Group, Inc., 1996.

Ballentine, Rudolph. *Transition to Vegetarianism.* Honesdale, PA: The Himalayan Institute Press, 1999.

Bender Birch, Beryl. *Beyond Power Yoga: 8 Levels of Practice for Body and Soul.* New York: Fireside, 2000.

———. *Power Yoga.* New York: Simon & Schuster, 1995.

Bhagavad Gita (multiple translations available).

Bouanchaud, Bernard. *The Essence of Yoga.* Portland: Rudra Press, 1997.

Bstan-'dzin-rgya-mtsho, Dalai Lama XIV (His Holiness the Dalai Lama). *The Art of Happiness.* New York: Riverhead Books, 1998.

———. *The Dalai Lama's Book of Wisdom.* New York: Thorsons Publishers, 2000.

———. *Healing Anger.* Ithaca, NY: Snow Lion Publications, 1997.

Budilovsky, Joan. *The Little Yogi Energy Book.* Oak Brook, IL: YOYOGA!, 1997.

———. *The Little Yogi Water Book.* Oak Brook, IL: YOYOGA!, 1998.

———. *Sun Salutations with Joan.* Oak Brook, IL: YOYOGA!, 1997.

———. *Yoga for a New Day.* Oak Brook, IL: YOYOGA!, 1996.

———. *Yoga with Joan.* Oak Brook, IL: YOYOGA!, 1996.

Budilovsky, Joan, and Eve Adamson. *The Complete Idiot's Guide to Massage.* Indianapolis: Alpha Books, 1998.

———. *The Complete Idiot's Guide to Meditation, Second Edition.* Indianapolis: Alpha Books, 2002.

Carper, Jean. *Jean Carper's Total Nutrition Guide.* New York: Bantam Books, 1987.

Chearney, Lee Ann. *Visits Caring for an Aging Parent: Reflections and Advice.* New York: Three Rivers Press, 1998.

Chopra, Deepak. *Ageless Body, Timeless Mind.* New York: Harmony Books, 1993.

Choudhury, Bikram. *Bikram's Beginning Yoga Class.* New York: G.P. Putnam's Sons, 2000.

Christensen, Alice. *The Easy Does It Yoga Trainer's Guide.* Sarasota, FL: American Yoga Association, 1995.

———. *Yoga of the Heart.* New York: Daybreak Books, 1998.

Cloutier, Marissa, M.S., R.D., Deborah S. Romaine, and Eve Adamson. *Beef Busters: Less Beef, Better Health!* Avon, MA: Adams Media Corporation, 2002.

Cloutier, Marissa, M.S., R.D., and Eve Adamson. *The Mediterranean Diet, Second Edition.* New York: HarperTouch, 2003.

Couch, Jean. *The Runner's Yoga Book.* Berkeley, CA: Rodmell Press, 1990.

de Mello, Anthony. *Wellsprings: A Book of Spiritual Exercises.* New York: Doubleday, 1984.

———. *Awareness: The Perils and Opportunities of Reality.* New York: Doubleday, 1992.

———. *Sadhana, A Way to God: Christian Exercises in Eastern Form.* New York: Doubleday, 1984.

Desikachar, T.K.V. *The Heart of Yoga: Developing a Personal Practice.* Rochester, VT: Inner Traditions International, 1995.

Dewey, John. *Experience and Education.* New York: Touchstone Edition, 1997.

Duff, Gail. *Eating Vegetarian: A Step-by-Step Guide.* Great Britain: Element Books Limited, 1999.

Farhi, Donna. *The Breathing Book: Good Health and Vitality Through Essential Breath Work.* New York: Henry Holt and Company, 1996.

Feuerstein, Georg. *The Shambhala Guide to Yoga*. Boston: Shambhala Publications, Inc., 1996.

———. *The Yoga Sutra of Patanjali: A New Translation and Commentary*. Rochester, VT: Inner Traditions, International, 1979.

Feuerstein, Georg, and Stephan Bodian, eds., with the staff of *Yoga Journal*. *Living Yoga: A Comprehensive Guide for Daily Life*. New York: Jeremy P. Tarcher/Perigee Books, 1993.

Flinders, Carol Lee. *At the Root of This Longing: Reconciling a Spiritual Hunger and a Feminist Thirst*. San Francisco: HarperSanFrancisco, 1998.

Flynn, Carolyn, and Erica Tismer. *Empowering Your Life with Massage*. Indianapolis: Alpha Books, 2004.

Flynn, Carolyn, and Shari Just. *The Complete Idiot's Guide to Creative Visualization*. Indianapolis: Alpha Books, 2005.

Francina, Suza. *The New Yoga for People Over 50*. Deerfield Beach, FL: Health Communications, Inc., 1997.

Franks, Samskrti, and Judith Franks. *Hatha Yoga Manual Two*. Honesdale, PA: The Himalayan International Institute, 1979.

Gandhi, Mahatma. *All Men Are Brothers*. India: Navajivan Publishing House, 1960.

Gandhi, Mohandask. *Gandhi's Health Guide*. Freedom, CA: The Crossing Press.

Gunther, Bernard. *Energy Ecstasy and Your Seven Vital Chakras*. North Hollywood, CA: Newcastle Publishing, 1983.

Hanh, Thich Nhat. *Peace Is Every Step*. New York: Bantam Books, 1991.

———. *The Miracle of Mindfulness*. Boston: Beacon Press, 1999.

Hanna, Thomas. *Somatics*. Reading, MA: Addison Wesley, 1988.

Harrar, Sari, and Sara Altshul O'Donnell. *The Woman's Book of Healing Herbs*. Emmaus, PA: Rodale Press, Inc., 1999.

Harvey, Andrew. *The Essential Mystics: The Soul's Journey into Truth*. San Francisco: HarperSanFrancisco, 1996.

Hess, Herbert J., and Charles O. Tucker. *Talking About Relationships*. Dubuque, IA: Kendall/Hunt, 1976.

Hewitt, James. *Teach Yourself Yoga*. Lincolnwood (Chicago), IL: NTC Publishing Group, 1993.

Hittleman, Richard. *Yoga for Health: The Total Program*. New York: Ballantine Books, 1983.

Iyengar, B.K.S. *Light on Yoga*. New York: Schocken Books, 1979.

———. *Yoga: The Path to Holistic Health*. New York: DK Publishing, 2001.

Japananda, Swami K. *Yoga, You, Your New Life*. Chicago: The Temple of Kriya Yoga, 1981.

Kabat-Zinn, Jon, Ph.D. *Full Catastrophe Living: Using the Wisdom of Your Body and Mind to Face Stress, Pain, and Illness*. New York: Delta, 1990.

Komitor, Jodi M., and Eve Adamson. *The Complete Idiot's Guide to Yoga with Kids*. Indianapolis: Alpha Books, 2000.

Kraftsow, Gary. *Yoga for Wellness*. New York: Penguin, 1999.

Kriyanada, Goswami. *Extraordinary Spiritual Potential*. Chicago: The Temple of Kriya Yoga, 1988.

———. *The Laws of Karma*. Chicago: The Temple of Kriya Yoga, 1995.

———. *The Spiritual Science of Kriya Yoga*. Chicago: The Temple of Kriya Yoga, 1992.

Kriyananda, Sri (J. Donald Walters). *Yoga Postures for Higher Awareness*. Nevada City, CA: Crystal Clarity, 1967.

Lasater, Judith, Ph.D. *Relax and Renew*. Berkeley, CA: Rodmell Press, 1995.

Lerner, Michael. *Choices in Healing: Integrating the Best of Conventional and Complementary Approaches to Cancer*. Cambridge, MA: MIT Press, 1994.

LeVert, Suzanne, and Gary McClain, Ph.D. *The Complete Idiot's Guide to Breaking Bad Habits, Second Edition*. Indianapolis: Alpha Books, 2001.

Levitt, Atma JoAnne. *The Kripalu Cookbook*. Stockbridge, MA: Berkshire House Publishers, 1995.

Mahabharata (numerous translations available).

Marshall, J. Dan, James T. Sears, and William J. Schubert. *Turning Points in Curriculum: A Contemporary American Memoir*. Upper Saddle River, NJ: Prentice Hall, 2000.

McClain, Gary R., Ph.D., and Eve Adamson. *The Complete Idiot's Guide to Zen Living, Second Edition*. Indianapolis: Alpha Books, 2004.

McHugh, Richard P., SJ., Ph.D. *Mind with a Heart*. India: Sadhana Institute, 1998.

McLaren, Karla. *Rebuilding the Garden*. Colum-bia, CA: Laughing Tree Press, 1997.

Mehta, Silva, and Shyam Mihra. *Yoga the Iyengar Way*. New York: A.A. Knopf, 1990.

Mishra, Rammurti S., M.D. *Fundamentals of Yoga*. New York: Harmony Books, 1987.

Monro, Robin, R. Nagaranthna, and H.R. Nagendra. *Yoga for Common Ailments*. New York: Fireside, 1990.

Moyers, Bill. *Healing and the Mind*. New York: Doubleday, 1993.

O'Brien, Paddy. *Yoga for Women: Complete Mind and Body Fitness*. London: Thorsons Publishers, 1994.

Paley, Vivian Gussin. *The Boy Who Would Be a Helicopter*. London: Harvard University Press, 1990.

Prabhupada, A.C., and Swami Bhaktivedanta. *Bhagavad-Gita as It Is*. Los Angeles: Bhaktivedanta Book Trust, 1968.

Rama, Swami. *Living with the Himalayan Masters*. Honesdale, PA: The Himalayan Institute Press, 1999.

———. *Path of Fire and Light*. Honesdale, PA: The Himalayan Institute Press, 1996.

Ramayana (numerous translations available).

Ravindra, Ravi. *Christ the Yogi*. Rochester, VT: Inner Traditions, 1998.

Rieker, Hans-Ulrich. *The Yoga of Light: Hatha Yoga Pradipika*. Middletown, CA: The Dawn House Press, 1971.

Rig Veda (multiple translations available).

Rush, Anne Kent. *The Modern Book of Yoga*. New York: Dell Publishing, 1996.

Satchidananda, Yogiraj Sri Swami. *Integral Yoga Hatha*. Satchidananda Ashram-Yogaville, VA: Integral Yoga Publications, 1998.

Scaravelli, Vanda. *Awakening the Spine*. New York: HarperCollins, 1991.

Schatz, Mary Pullig, M.D. *Back Care Basics*. Berkeley, CA: Rodmell Press, 1992.

Schiffmann, Erich. *Yoga: The Spirit and Practice of Moving Into Stillness*. New York: Pocket Books, 1996.

Sivananda Yoga Vedanta Center. *Learn Yoga in a Weekend*. New York: Alfred A. Knopf, 1995.

————. *The Sivananda Companion to Yoga*. New York: Simon & Schuster, 1983.

————. *Yoga Mind Body*. New York: DK Publishing, 1996.

Somar, Sonia. *Yoga for the Special Child*. Buckingham, VA: Special Yoga Publications, 1998.

Stewart, Mary, and Kathy Phillips. *Yoga for Children*. London: Webster's International Publishers, 1992.

Stroud, Francis J., S.J., *Praying Naked, The Spirituality of Anthony de Mello*. New York, Doubleday, 2005.

Takoma, Geo, and Eve Adamson. *The Complete Idiot's Guide to Power Yoga*. Indianapolis: Alpha Books, 1999.

Tigunait, Pandit Rajmani. *Inner Quest: The Path of Spiritual Unfoldment*. Honesdale, PA: Yoga International Books, 1995.

Upanishads (multiple translations available).

Vishnudevananda, Swami. *The Complete Illustrated Book of Yoga*. New York: Bell Publishers, 1960.

Yogananda, Paramahansa. *Autobiography of a Yogi*. Los Angeles: Self-Realization Fellowship, 1946.

————. *God Talks with Arjuna*. Los Angeles: Self-Realization Fellowship, 2004.

————. *Journey to Self-Realization: Discovering the Gifts of the Soul*. Los Angeles: Self-Realization Fellowship, 1997.

————. *The Second Coming of Christ: The Resurrection of Christ Within You*. Los Angeles: Self-Realization Fellowship, 2004.

Yogi Bhajan, Ph.D. *Kundalini Yoga: The Flow of Eternal Power*. Los Angeles: Time Capsule Books, 1996.

Yukteswar, Swami Sri. *The Holy Science*. Los Angeles: Self-Realization Fellowship, 1949.

Index

I

More Books and Tapes by Joan Budilovsky

Special Offer for Readers of
The Complete Idiot's Guide to Yoga Illustrated, Fourth Edition

Joan's CDs, Tapes, and Books

Yoga Audio

	CD	Cassette
Yoga with Joan One hour of meditative postures and breathwork.	$12.00	$10.00
Breathworks! Thirty minutes of deep-breathing exercises.	$12.00	$10.00
Sun-Salutations! with Joan A dynamic series of yoga postures with meditation exercises.	$12.00	$10.00
Total Relaxation with Shavasana Shavasana + meditation = BLISS.	$12.00	$10.00
Beach Blanket Yoga Thirty minutes of yoga fun in the sun.	N/A	$10.00
Body and Soul Meditation Harp music, Joan's voice, and you.	$12.00	N/A

Massage Audio

	CD	Cassette
The Art of Massage Made Simple Joan guides you in giving a one-hour full-body Swedish massage.	$12.00	$10.00
Foot Massage for Body, Mind, and Sole Relax your feet. Relax your whole body.	$12.00	$10.00

Massage Video

	DVD	Video
My Swedish Massage with Joan Instructional video on many of the massage strokes featured in *The Complete Idiot's Guide to Massage.*	15.00	$15.00

Mini Yoga Books

	Book
The Little Yogi Energy Book Small but powerful! Energize yourself with these terrific chakra postures.	$10.00
The Little Yogi Water Book Yoga poses done in water with a partner.	$10.00
Yoga for a New Day Compact yoga lifestyle guides with simple postures.	$10.00

Come visit Joan at her Yoyoga! website: www.yoyoga.com

Order form on NEXT PAGE

Yes, send me copies of Joan's wonderful tapes and books.

Yoga Audio		CD	Cassette
❑ *Yoga with Joan*		$12.00	$10.00
❑ *Breathworks!*		$12.00	$10.00
❑ *Sun-Salutations! with Joan*		$12.00	$10.00
❑ *Total Relaxation with Shavasana*		$12.00	$10.00
❑ *Beach Blanket Yoga*		N/A	10.00
❑ *Body and Soul Meditation*		$12.00	N/A

Massage Audio		CD	Cassette
❑ *The Art of Massage Made Simple*		$12.00	$10.00
❑ *Foot Massage for Body, Mind, and Sole*		$12.00	$10.00

Massage		DVD	Video
❑ *My Swedish Massage with Joan*		$15.00	$15.00

Mini Yoga Books	Book
❑ *The Little Yogi Energy Book*	$10.00
❑ *The Little Yogi Water Book*	$10.00
❑ *Yoga for a New Day*	$10.00

Shipping/handling charges:

Audio/book	Add $2.50 for one or two items; add $.50 for each additional item.	$_____
Video	Add $4.50 for first videotape; add $1.00 for each additional videotape.	$_____
	Subtotal	$_____
	Illinois residents add 6.75% sales tax	$_____
	Outside United States additional $5.00 to subtotal	$_____
	TOTAL	$_____

Payment to be made in U.S. funds. Prices and availability are subject to change without notice.
❑ Check or money order enclosed.
❑ I would like to charge to: ❑ MasterCard   ❑ Visa

Acct. #: _____

Exp. Date: _____

Signature: _____

Send this order form with your check, money order, or charge information to:

Yoyoga, Inc.
P.O. Box 5013
Oak Brook, IL 60522
Phone: 630-587-YOGA (9642)
Fax: 630-587-9645

Allow four to six weeks for delivery.

Ship to:

Name: _____

Address: _____

City, State, Zip: _____

Telephone: _____